Avatar's Prescription

*Stories of medical service and guidance received
from Bhagawan Sri Sathya Sai Baba*

Dr. M. Vijai Kumar M.D., D.A.

Copies of book available at: Publications Division -
Sri Sathya Sai Sadhana Trust, Prashanthi Nilayam

© Dr. M. Vijai Kumar 2017

All Rights Reserved

The copyright and the rights of translation in any language are reserved by the Author and publisher. No part, para, passage, text, photograph, or Art work of this Book should be reproduced, transmitted or utilized, in original language or by translation, in any form or by any means, electronic, mechanical, photo copying, recording, or by any information, storage and retrieval system, except with prior permission, in writing from the author, except for brief passages quoted in book review.

International Standard Book Number: 978-164008391-2

First Edition: July 2017

Published by:
Dr. M. Vijai Kumar M.D., D.A.
Sai Prema, 4/14 East Avenue,
Kesavaperumal Puram, Chennai 600 028.
India
drvijaikumar@gmail.com

Printed at:
SVL Ltd.
Gummidipoondi,
Thiruvallur District - 601 201.
India

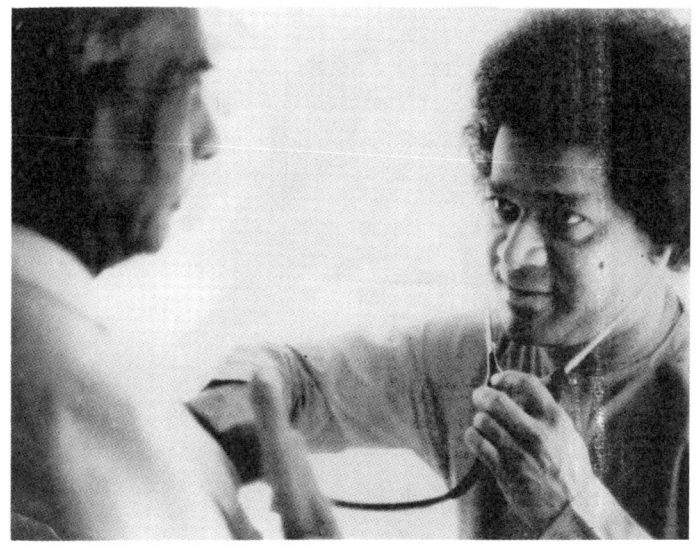

Iconic picture of Bhagawan Sri Sathya Sai Baba examining Dr. Sunder Rao of Bangalore. Attention and empathy are wonderful tools for giving care… and here's Bhagawan modelling these tools for all of us.

Foreword

Om Sai Ram!

It's a great privelage and pleasure for me to write a foreword for this wonderful book on our beloved Swami written by my collegue and dear friend Dr. M. Vijai Kumar. I have known Dr. Vijai Kumar for several years, first as a professional collegue(being a fellow doctor), later in connection with SaiKrupa activities, and still later as a fellow trustee of Sri Sathya Sai Trust, Tamil Nadu.

Dr. Vijai Kumar is one of the senior most devotees of Swami amongst the members of medical profession in Tamil Nadu. This book written by him contains invaluable nuggets of Dr. Vijai Kumar's association with our beloved Swami. Written in a easy to read style, filled with love, affection, and devotion for Bhagawan Sri Sathya Sai Baba. The book is a veritable feast not only for Sai devotees but for everyone. Dr. Vijai Kumar has carefully chronicled his various interactions with Swami. He also honestly and beautifully describes various miracles and they range from his experiences as a devotee, as a member of Sai organization, as medical doctor in SaiKrupa, to his speciality of anesthesia and the lesson he learned "inside the operating theatre". He also talks about Swami's various projects such as Sathya Sai Healthcare projects including the SaiKrupas at Chennai, and at Prashanthi Nilayam and Whitefield, international medical conference at Prashanthi Nilayam, mother and child program at Prashanthi Nilayam, the autorickshaw drivers diabetic camps, eye camps, organized at Chennai.

All in all, for all those who are interested in learning first hand a medical doctor's experiences, and to learn about the glory about our beloved Bhagawan through the personal experiences of one of his ardent devotees, this book would be the one to read and treasure. I cannot but admire Dr. Vijai Kumar for his passion and devotion to Swami. I know how difficult it is to write a book of this nature but Dr. Vijai Kumar has done it elegantly and with ease, obviously inspired by, and blessed by, Bhagawan Baba. I am extremely grateful to him for having requested me to write a foreword for his book. I hope to see the book in print soon and wish and pray that it is read by thousands of people who, I am sure, will be inspired by various incidents narrated in this book.

Dr. V. Mohan

Dr. V. Mohan M.D., FRCP(London, Edin, Glas, Ireland), Ph.D., DSc., DSc. (Hon. Causa), FNASc., FASc., FNA, FACP, FACE, FTWAS

Trustee, Sri Sathya Sai Central Trust, Prasanthi Nilayam
Convener, Sri Sathya Sai Trust, Tamilnadu

Chairman, Dr. Mohan's Diabetes Specialities Center
President, Madras Diabetes Research Foundation
Awarded Padma Shri by President of India
Dr. B. C. Roy Award by Medical Council of India

Foreword

Om Sai Ram!

Few physicians in this world have been blessed with such close association and direct guidance from Sathya Sai Baba over so many years as Dr. Vijai Kumar of Chennai, India. I had the good fortune of meeting Dr. Vijai Kumar and his wife - Mrs. Dakshayani - several years ago at my home, along with his daughter Aparna Murali and his son Sanjai Murali, whom I had know for many years. We soon learned of our mutual interest in providing medical services in free medical clinics and camps.

In this book, Dr. Kumar describes his many interactions with Sri Sathya Sai Baba and the direct suggestions and instructions he received on organizing and carrying out service projects to benefit society. The scope, variety, and impact of the service projects are awe inspiring, ranging from free medical clinics and camps to the massive Water Project in Chennai, which provided pure and free water to more than 8 million people who had been suffering for decades from lack of water. The personal story of how his devotion to Swami and His teachings transformed him as a person, physician, and anesthesiologist is equally compelling. Dr. Kumar is a role model par excellence for medical providers as well as for anyone aspiring to be a good human being. He demonstrates, through the service projects described, that when we look for opportunities to serve others, we will surely discover many opportunities to help, and that to start such good works, money is not a prerequisite. Dr. Kumar's narrative is augmented with wonderful pictures illustrating the numerous service projects he had the fortune to be involved with and capturing the feelings of joy both in those who received the services and those who provided them.

As an example, Dr. Kumar once noticed long lines of patients waiting to receive various services at the general hospital he worked at in Chennai, and identified an opportunity to help. A team was then formed to direct the daily crowds of 8,000 to 10,000 patients, who often waited in the wrong line, into organized and efficient lines to feed to all departments. The team of approximately 15 volunteers also provided water, wheelchair assistance, Telugu interpreting services, and other services as needed. These volunteers, identifiable by their orange scarves, helped transform the chaos, frustration, and long waits into order and peace of mind. This brilliant story of innovative and loving crowd control illustrates how thousands of patients were helped to get the services they needed in an efficient manner, while also helping the physicians and staff in the hospital to provide those services in a more optimum way.

Dr. Kumar also shares numerous pearls of wisdom from Sathya Sai Baba, applicable to all medical practitioners, medical students, and service volunteers. Some of these include:

> *Kindness and compassion are tools you should use in your practice. Half of your patients' problems will be resolved by your empathy, and never take undue risks. You should ask yourself, would you attempt the same if the patient were your kith and kin?*
>
> *Look with eyes of compassion, and opportunities for service will stare at you.*
>
> *You should be careful to pay great attention to every little detail in any project you are doing, focus on the present, and do your absolute best for every small, medium, or large task.*

I was inspired and humbled by these stories of medical service; once I started reading, it was hard to stop before finishing the entire book. The divine guidance Dr. Kumar received and the heartwarming stories of the amazing medical service projects he participated in will certainly be referred to for generations to come. Each person who reads this book will come away with a perspective on how much is possible when we have good intentions to help others and the courage to take action. Especially inspiring were the medical camps serving children with post-polio disability, who received compassionate care and also state of the art medical care via surgery, calipers, and braces to help them regain the ability to walk with crutches. The volunteers were witness to these children's smiling faces as they walked again for the first time in years.

With all the negativity we see in the media and news today, it is helpful and reassuring to learn of pure-hearted individuals like Dr. Kumar and the many volunteers in the Sathya Sai Seva Organization in Tamil Nadu, India, who take advantage of every opportunity to help and who use their knowledge and skills to serve others. An important message also becomes evident regarding the power of good intentions. When someone notices suffering and has pure intentions to help, God will provide all the resources necessary to accomplish this task. All this can be done without public fundraising, allowing the sole focus to be on rendering loving and compassionate service to those in need. How this happens is described compellingly in the beautiful stories in this book, and I have witnessed the same phenomenon with my own eyes in many other service projects in India, the USA, and other countries.

Readers stand to realize the golden opportunity we all have to use our knowledge and skills to help others. It is hoped that through imbibing these stories, all will be inspired to take action in their local communities with renewed vigor and enthusiasm.

Joseph G. Phaneuf M.D.

Chairman, USA Medical Committee, Sathya Sai International Organization (SSIO);

Medical Director, Ashland Free Medical Clinic, San Lorenzo, CA, USA

(first SSSIO Medical Clinic in the USA, in operation since January 8, 2005);

National Advisor, Young Adult Program, SSSIO, USA

Dedication

Bhagawan says "Swami Premanu Panchuko, Penchuko"– share Swami's love and make it grow. Bhagawan has blessed me to be involved in "medical seva" for more than 4 ½ decades. Swami has taught me many lessons through varied experiences which form the narrative for this book. Some biographical events and details have also been included because of lessons learnt and the desire that it may be of use to fellow pilgrims who may be in similar situations and asking similar questions. Swami's teachings are timeless and essential and applicable for all. As early as the 1950s, in a young nation albeit a old country, Bhagawan Sri Sathya Sai Baba laid the foundation for the General Hospital at Puttaparthi. Puttaparthi, an obscure village in the hinterland then, had no access to medical facilities unless one undertakes a long and arduous journey to closest urban area of Bangalore. With this act, the Avatar, quietly and without much fanfare, ushered in an paradigm of medical care, that is marvelled today by nation states across the world, including the World Health Organization(WHO).

Bhagawan's medical mission had started – not only to serve the needy in the village of Puttaparthi, but to also serve as a model, a template for medical care, for all of humanity. In the 21st century, the gulf between the haves and have-nots has widened beyond measure. This gulf is plain and apparent when it comes to accessing life saving medical services. Whilst the rich afford state of art care, the poor run from pillar to post to fend off fate's fury. Rich or poor, democratic or autocratic, socialist or capitalist, irrespective of political and philosophical persuasion, governments the world over are grappling with how to provide medical care that doesn't leave behind the poor while balancing books of the state.

Bhagawan's medical mission stands tall as a beacon of light in a sea of darkness, guiding humanity that is on the verge of destroying the seams that hold its constituent parts together. At its heart, Bhagawan's medical mission is based on love and compassion, not on balancing books or principles of commerce. He has stated categorically time and again, that a fundamental need as medical care must be offered free to members of society, irrespective of their socio-economic status. SaiKrupa, a free outpatient clinic, started in Chennai in 1979, at Bhagawan's command, serves as a model to humanity – to provide free medical care to one and all. SaiKrupa like free clinics have spread not only in Tamil Nadu but all over the world. Bhagawan's personal involvement in initiating and nurturing SaiKrupa, His divine counsel to doctors and sevadals on how to provide medical care, is chronicled in the stories and anecdotes that constitute Avatar's Prescription which is held by your hands. To borrow the words of Prof. Kasturi, the first biographer of Bhagawan, these are stories that illumine in a flash on what medical care is all about, these are stories that correct our collective astigmatic vision of medical care, most of all these are stories that give us insight on Avatar's tireless labour of love to set medical care - a key pillar of society – on a firm foundation of love and compassion.

Avatars come to accomplish grand tasks. The very first cities on Earth were established by Prithu – an Avatar of lord Vishnu. The very first super speciality Hospital with free care was established by the Avatar of the age - Bhagawan Sri Sathya Sai Baba. This epoch making event is sure to cause ripple effects for eternity. In His immense love for humanity, Bhagawan has not only given us a prescription for medical care, He has also mercifully shown us - through His life - how to fulfil this prescription.

The author humbly offers this book at Bhagawan's lotus feet, with a prayer that all of us must fulfil Avatar's Prescription and make medical care available to all, irrespective of one's socio-economic status.

Jai Sairam!

Dr. M. Vijai Kumar

Table of Contents

Foreword by Dr. V. Mohan	i
Foreword by Dr. Joseph Phaneuf	iii
Dedication	vii

Section 1 – Early Days 1

Historical Perspective	3
Planting Seeds	6
First Sai Eye Camp in Tamil Nadu	8
Unity & Enthusiasm Draws God	10
Don't Need Brains to Experience Love	12
Transformation in Tondiarpet Home	14
School Health Checkup Scheme	16
From Chaos to Order and Harmony	18
Blood Donation Campaign	20
24x7 Blood Donation Service at Sundaram	22
Relay Medical Service – Story of Joseph	23
Sai Supports	25
Hands that Help are Holier than Lips that Pray	27
Sai Free Clinics in the City	30
Birth of SaiKrupa	35
Medicine Bank	37
Sookshma Sai Clinical Lab	39
Sai Niketan	40
Sathya Sai Mission Hospital – Coimbatore	42
Happy Home at Poondamalli	44

Section 2 – Expanding Medical Service 47

Bhagawan's Visit to SaiKrupa..	49
Abbotsbury Transforms into Eye Hospital............................	52
Spare 2 Tablets for My Grace..	57
Bringing Care to Senior Citizens...	61
All India Seva Training – Prashanthi Nilayam......................	64
Bhagawan's Advice on Eye Camps..	65
They Wanted to do All the Walking......................................	66
Dental Camp..	73
WHO Team Visits SaiKrupa...	74
Silver Jubilee of Sai Organization...	75
SaiKrupa on the Move...	77
Antony From Anatomy Lab...	79
Bhagawan's Blessings to Doctors..	80
Love is Expansion...	83
Medical Seva at Prashanthi and Whitefield...........................	84
Health Meters for Auto Drivers...	86
Humanising Medicare..	89
Sri Sathya Sai Healthcare Project (2007)..............................	90
Sri Sathya Sai Total Healthcare – A Working Model............	92
SaiKrupa Events..	93

Section 3 – Personal Experiences 97

First Encounter: Earliest Prescriptions..................................	98
Cases Referred by Bhagawan..	102
Bhagawan and a Patient..	106

Journey via Anesthesia Practice	109
Lessons Inside Operating Theatre	111
Smile and be Always Reassuring	113
Bhagawan's Ways are Mysterious	114
Career Guidance	116
A Course in Engineering and Management for a Doctor	118
Chennai Water Project	120
Red Maruti Car	122
No Garlands for Me?	125
Prescriptions Received During Darshan	127
Dorikindhi Dachuko	128
This is also a form of Devotion	130
Seva and Service	131
You Do My Work, I'll Do Your Work	134
Divine Permission	136
Visiting Cards and Gifts of Love	137
Gratitude	140
Epilogue	142

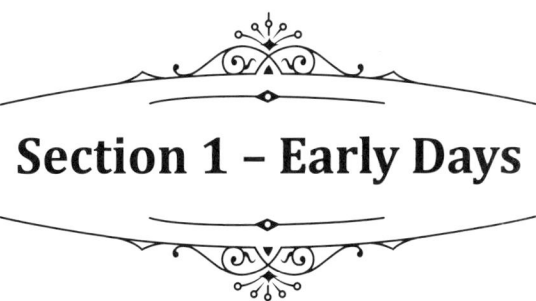

Section 1 – Early Days

Historical Perspective

During Lord Rama's time – which according to Bhagawan was 10,000 odd years ago – we know of the battlefield injury sustained by His brother Lakshmana that caused him to faint. Hanuman was able to recruit the renowned physician of those times – Sushena – to help diagnose the condition of Lakshmana who was unconscious. Sushena prescribed the miracle herb sanjeevani to revive Lakshmana. The only problem: this herb was available in the foothills of Himalayas, thousands of miles north of the battlefield. Being endowed with the power to fly at will, Hanuman air dashed to Himalayas. Not knowing which herb to pick in the midst of several similar looking herbs, Hanuman plucked an entire mountain of the ground and airlifted it to the battlefield. Sushena was able to spot the required sanjeevani herb and thus revive Lakshmana. Hanuman was probably a precursor to modern day air ambulances – choppers fitted with life saving equipment and drugs and manned by experts in emergency medicine. Care was provisioned where it was needed the most – healthcare system shouldn't impose the burden of finding care on those in dire need. This is a timeless lesson for everyone in the healthcare ecosystem and one brought to light frequently by Bhagawan. The mobile hospital commissioned by Bhagawan which serves many hamlets and villages in the vicinity of Parthi serves exactly this purpose of bringing care to the door step of those in need.

In the 5th century before Christ, Herodotus of Greece, documents a social form of healthcare delivery that was ordained by the King of the land. Those who were diseased were admitted to a public square, where every passer-by had to perforce stop and have a conversation with the diseased. If they had suffered the same condition, they had to share the remedy. If they had known anyone who had suffered the same condition, they had to share which remedy had worked successfully. Even if the passer-by had not suffered the same condition or known anyone who suffered the same and had a remedy, he or she had to perforce converse with the diseased. Medicine was a not a well developed branch of science in the western world, and the system of care had to make do with the public knowledge of remedy. The public square was a precursor to the modern day hospital system, which is said to be the work of Romans.

The larger lesson is that everyone has a role to play in healthcare… the rulers of today do not mandate that we stop by at the public square of our times – Hospitals – and enquire about the condition of every patient. In some countries such as USA, there are privacy regulations that prohibit a patient's condition from being known publicly. The population of Greece in 5th century BC made the model of public square possible then. Modern day social networks are beginning to play this role. 'Patientslikeme.com' is a case in point. Physician network, epocrates.com, allows physicians to share remedies and knowledge they have gained with other physicians. One needn't be a physician to play a role in healthcare of one's community and society. Disseminating health and hygiene information, providing support services at point of care, providing caring companionship, and above all, sharing a kind word and a smile goes a long way in healing and recovery. These are areas where Sai organization, under Bhagawan's loving guidance, has been providing yeoman services to the world - filling a critical gap in Healthcare on a global scale. To my knowledge, no other organization provides the breadth of healthcare services, free of cost, as does the Sai Organization.

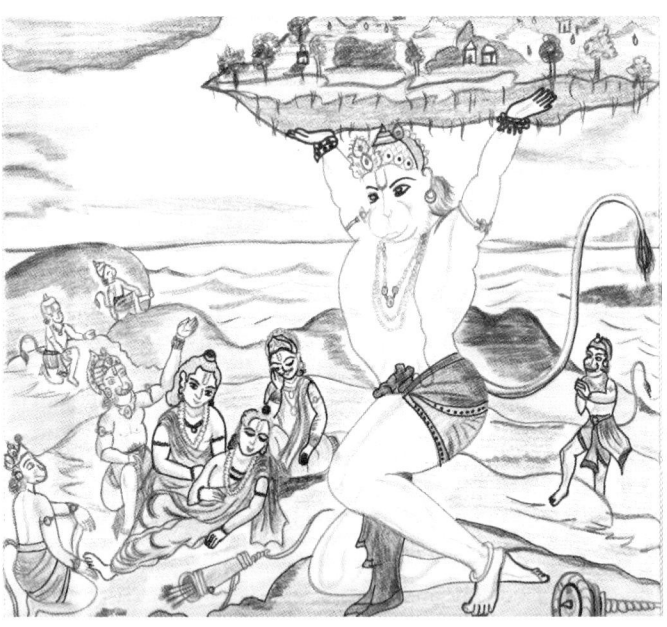

Hanuman airlifts a mountain containing the Sanjeevani herb to the battlefield in Lanka (modern day Sri Lanka), to aid recovery of Lakshmana-brother of Lord Rama

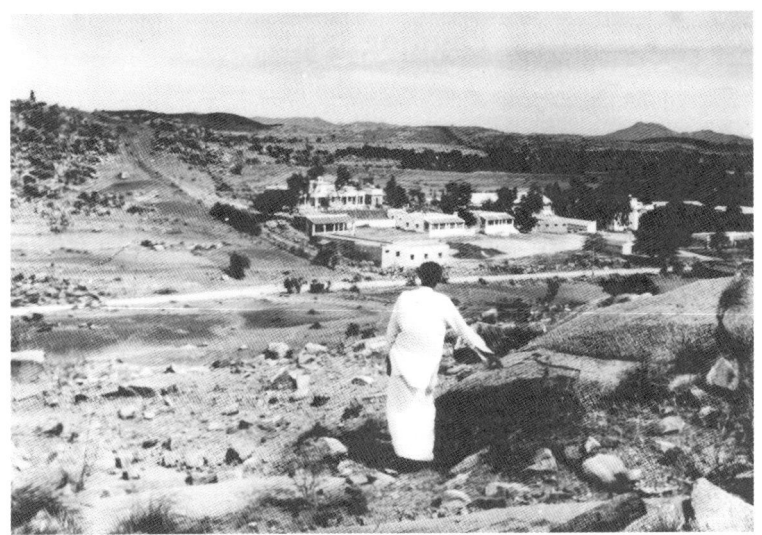

General Hospital nestled in the hills of Puttaparthi as seen in late 1950's - seen farthest from the man standing is the General Hospital building. The twin buildings in the foreground comprised Veda Pata Shala block. Back of the Prashanthi Mandir can be seen far right of the twin buildings

Planting Seeds

Who can fathom what lies in the womb of time? Bhagawan once told a devotee: "whereas you plan for your children and grand children, I plan for many many generations". Such is the expansive vision of Bhagawan.

It was the first anniversary of Podanur (suburb of Coimbatore) Samithi. Bhagawan had deputed Sri. N. Kasturi to preside and participate in the celebrations. Sri. Kasturi delivered a discourse for nearly four hours on "108 Padams" - one hundred and eight stories depicting glory of Swami's lotus feet. Inspired by this, I joined the Sathya Sai Organization as a member of Podanur Samithi in 1970. I also attended bhajans at Coimbatore Samithi. It was at Coimbatore Samithi where I met Dr. P. Punnaivanam - a general practioner who was running a free Sai clinic at Ram Nagar bhajan unit. He used to attend on 30 to 40 patients for about an hour before the weekly bhajans. He was a busy practitioner and at the same time very much service minded. In those days, he was the only doctor available for about sixteen hamlets and villages in and around Ondipudur(near Coimbatore). I once accompanied him on his village rounds – this included driving his car for 8 km in unpaved dirt road, running half a kilometer through a pathway where he couldn't drive the car, in order to attend on a child having convulsion. He administered an injection and returned without collecting any fee from the poor farmer. All the villagers had great love and respect for him. Witnessing selfless service and its outcome was a great source of inspiration. Thus Bhagawan planted the seeds of medical service in my heart.

On one occasion, I was traveling with Dr. Punnaivanam in his car. He suddenly pulled over near a thatched tea stall on the village road. From behind the hut, I saw two people carrying a patient on a coir cot. Dr. Punnaivanam got down took a syringe from his box, loaded the medicine, and administered the same, and then resumed driving – in less than a minute. He explained that the patient was suffering from TB; he was administering the streptomycin injection, daily. He also explained how he had organized two volunteers to carry the poor patient to the road side so that he could administer the injection on his morning round of villages. He also explained how the volunteers would carry the patient back and stop at two rich farmers' houses on the way. The doctor had arranged for a cup of milk at house no.1 and for a raw egg to be poured directly in the mouth of the patient in the house no.2 - thus not only the treatment but also the nutrition for the patient was looked after. He did not stop with that. He arranged a temporary job in a Ginning factory for his wife, so that the family does not starve during the patient's recovery period of three months. Even the labour unions did not object to this out of turn employment because it was on the good doctor's recommendation. I was stunned to find how nicely Dr. Punnaivanam had worked out the total treatment, nutrition, and rehabilitation of the poor villager. It is said, "Vaidyo Naryano Hari" - doctor is none other than the Lord himself. It wasn't surprising to see villagers revere Dr. Punnaivanam as God Himself.

This kind of silent Sai Seva was being carried out by Dr. Punnaivanam. From a member of Coimbatore Samithi, he rose to become state Sevadal convenor. Bhagawan graciously appointed him as a member of council of management, Sri Sathya Sai Trust, Tamil Nadu.

For every major seva project, Dr. Punnaivanam used to seek Bhagawan's blessings. On one occasion, Bhagawan assured him saying "when you perform seva with a pure heart, a blank cheque is given to you. You can draw any amount of grace!".

I am deeply grateful for the inspiration given by Bhagawan through Dr. Punnaivanam. Unbeknown to me, this inspiration prepared the ground and sowed the seeds for a future harvest…who can plan with such foresight? Only Bhagawan can – the cultivator par excellence.

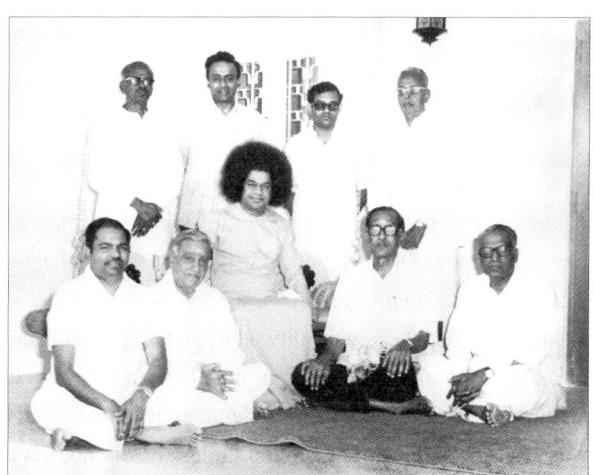

Dr. Punnaivanam seen seated extreme left, as Bhagawan poses with His Tamil Nadu Trust members(Sathya Sai Trust) – Circa late 1970's. Standing left to right: Sri. P.G. Achuthanantham, Sri. V. Srinivasan, Sri. Sachithanandam, Sri. Ramanathan Chettiar. Sitting to left of Dr. Punnaivanam: Sri. Damodar Rao, Maj. Rayningar, Sri. Manickyavachagam

First Sai Eye Camp in Tamil Nadu

Any selfless thought to benefit humanity becomes a recipient of Bhagawan's grace. During second half of 1970, Dr. Punnaivanam came up with the idea to conduct an eye camp as a "service project". A classmate of Dr. Punnaivanam, an Ophthalmologist practicing in Coimbatore came forward to screen patients and operate on Cataract cases free of charge. Dr. Punnaivanam offered his small nursing home used mainly for maternity cases – consisting of 6 beds - for about a week, to be used for eye camp. Being an anesthesiologist by training, I took on the task of scrubbing the operation theatre and sterilizing the same for eye surgery. Wide publicity was given in the neighbouring villages. On day one, the screening and selection of fit cases for surgery was done. Entire Sai Organization was involved on day one during screening and day two during surgery, Bhajans were being sung continuously in a shamiana erected in the compound. From about 80 patients who attended the screening, 8 were selected for surgery. The next step was what was called a "trial bandage". The eye to be operated would be thoroughly washed and then kept closed over night by applying a pad and a bandage. The following morning, eyes are examined. Any redness means lurking infection and so unfit for operation. Those were the days when powerful antibiotics were not available. Thus out of the 8 selected patients, two became unfit for surgery.

Preparations were getting ready for surgery when one of the six patients found fit, declared that he did not want surgery. Everyone felt disappointed as he walked out after refusing surgery. Just at that moment a new patient walked in and wanted to know whether he could be operated. It was God sent substitute for the one who walked away. This gentleman was obese and could lie down flat with great difficulty. But the doctors accepted him as things were ready for six cases. The surgery started as planned. One by one, the patients were wheeled out of the operating theatre into their own rooms for a weeks stay. Meticulous instructions were given and the camp had the luxury of two volunteers attending on each patient round the clock. After thorough preparation, the obese patient was taken up last. Inspite of adequate sedation he was moving his head frequently. The local anaesthesia was effective and acting well and though he did not have any pain he was very un-cooperative. During the post-operative period he tried to pull off the bandage twice. All the doctors were skeptical about the outcome in his case.

Duty roster had been drawn up and home cooked food was prepared for the patients. A devotee couple would come and feed the patients and look after them until the next batch reported. Breakfast, lunch, and dinner were thus organized for all the seven days. Daily morning and evening, there would be bhajans for the welfare of the patients.

Morning of 8th day, bandage was opened and each patient advised to slowly open the operated eye before a huge picture of Swami. Each patient would have their first darshan with the regained vision. All patients were supplied with glasses along with Swami's prasadam.

All patients had gained perfect vision in the operated eye. There were traces of redness due to inflammation in a couple of patients. Our last obese patient was the happiest and he did not have even a trace of redness in his operated eye inspite of all that had happened. Everyone was stunned to see the result in this patient. It was sheer Sai grace. Anything done with pure love and sincerity always has the umbrella of Divine protection.

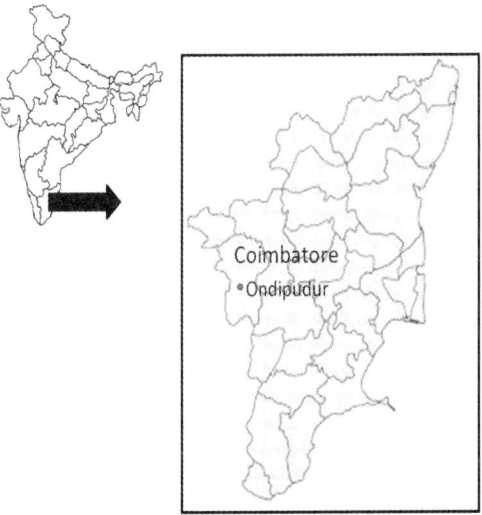

The first Sai eye camp was conducted in 1970 in Ondipudur, Coimbatore. Patients from rural areas benefitted from this eye camp.

It was an eye camp in many dimensions. Whilst patients were blessed with clear vision following successful cataract surgeries, doctors and sevadals were blessed with a clear vision of how to conduct future medical camps.

> When the eye has a cataract over the pupil, one can't see anything at all. So too, when the notion of the body being the reality is predominant, the resident in the body isn't noticed at all." - Baba

Unity & Enthusiasm Draws God

Encouraged by the experience of the first eye camp, volunteers were very enthusiastic about organizing a community service on a holiday. Thus, the idea was born to pool resources and offer a major general medical camp in a rural set-up. It is said that when men come together in a spirit of enthusiasm and unity, God becomes a willing accomplice. How this accomplice manifested himself is a tale of grace. At this time, another active worker from Coimbatore Samithi, Sri. Venkatraman joined the planning team. He was working at Soolur Airforce Station(near Coimbatore) at that time. Dr. Punnaivanam and I were inspired by him as he infused ideas of meticulous and detailed planning – provision of back-up for contingencies, handling of crowds, logistics and allocation of work-force etc. were included with the thoroughness of the Armed forces. A "winding up team" was an idea born out of this method of planning. Generally, whenever a major event is planned, enthusiasm wanes due to exhaustion towards the end of the program. A fresh team of work force is kept in readiness to wind up, clean the place and handover in a spic and span condition. Today, this practice has become a standard and is part of Sai events. However, in those early days of medical service, this was a new concept – that it was readily embraced and adopted by volunteers speaks about the spirit of unity, and the spirit of Sai that permeated through all volunteers.

Dr. Punnaivanam was a visiting doctor for various textile mills in the periphery of the city, therefore it was easy for him to get a place for the Sunday medical camp in the campus of one of the mills. I must acknowledge the managers of these mills who went out of their way to provide facilities like – shamianas, furniture, temporary power and water connections, food arrangements, etc. I was tasked with planning the technical aspects of arranging medical man power and procuring equipment for their use in the camp. I was working at the E.S.I. Hospital at Varadarajapuram, and could therefore enlist the services of all the specialists for the camp. Thus the first general medical camp was organized in a textile mill campus with nearly 200 volunteers participating along with 50 doctors in a rural setup under the Sai Organization banner.

Publicity was given by local announcement in the villages, pamphlet distribution and door to door canvassing for chronic patients to make use of the camp and giving them registration slips with camp details. About 1600 patients availed the services provided in the camp. It was amazing to see voluntary offers in kind pouring in, such as rice bags, milk, vegetables etc. Everybody was overjoyed to participate in the event. Love begets Love. Sai grace was felt in abundance during the entire camp with continuous bhajans being sung during the camp.

There were so many willing accomplices who aided and abetted this medical camp – Sri. Venkatraman who brought the discipline and detail of planning from Armed Forces, the managers at the textile mill who wholeheartedly opened their campus and provided logistics support, the many specialists who willingly came to serve on a Sunday, many who voluntarily contributed in kind, and devotees who volunteered with enthusiasm. It would be naïve to think we did it – it was Sai who orchestrated the whole event and conferred on us the joy of being His instruments.

Don't Need Brains to Experience Love

During June 1973, I had to move to Madras(now Chennai) due to work. By Swami's grace I was selected to undergo "in service training" in M.D. Anesthesiology at M.M.C. and Govt. General Hospital, Madras. Sri P.G. Achuthanantham, then State President of B.S.S.S.O of Tamil Nadu got me enrolled as Madras Samithi member. In those days, membership in Sai Samithi wasn't automatic. Each membership had to be approved by local Sai organization and for some time, Swami Himself would approve the list of devotees who are to be granted membership. Digression complete, let me bring you back to the story. Sri. Achuthanantham had attended Coimbatore Eye Camp and so he wanted me to start medical service activities at Madras also. He actually took me to two orphanages in the city and wanted me to attend on the children for their medical needs. One was "Sisu Bhavan" - a home for unwanted children run by Mother Theresa at Royapuram and another was an orphanage at Tondairpet, where children who commit petty crimes and wander the streets are committed to this home by the police. This home had children below 12 years and had a primary school attached to it. Both the places offered formidable challenges and I started visiting both the homes on Thursday afternoon every week to offer medical seva.

At Sisu Bhavan, there was no dearth for funds. The sisters were able to buy prescribed medicine and look after the patients with love. They had a system by which they would leave a empty cradle in a shaded place in the compound and leave the gates unlocked for the night. Every morning the sister will inspect the cradle and pick up children (unwanted) left by parents in the darkness of the dawn. They would attend to them with love and bring them up. They would request me to name them during the Thursday visit. I used to choose Hindu, Muslim and Christian names by turns and the sisters would gladly register them as such. The healthy children would go for adoption. Those days the rules were not so stringent. Sishu Bhavan used to be left with retarded children - children with congenital defects and palsies. It was an amazing experience for me to see the sisters attending on these children with so much love.

I want to share my experience with one of the inmates – Sheela, who was about eight to ten years old. Physically her growth was like any other normal child but her head was the size of a small coconut or a large lime. She could walk and move about by herself and respond to small commands. She used to develop frequent convulsions and whatever brain power was left in that small skull, was further reduced by the heavy sedatives she was receiving as medication for her convulsions. Sisters had to feed her and attend to her personal hygiene. Sheela took a great liking for me. She would catch hold of my little finger, cling to me, accompany me on my rounds and then leave me at the gate. Sheela could not talk or communicate in anyway but there developed a strong bond between me and this child -Sheela. If for some reasons, I missed visiting Sishu Bhavan, the following week the Sister was sure to say " Doctor, you did not come last Thursday. Sheela was waiting for you at the gate from 2.00 p.m. onwards". It was strange that Sheela who had zero I.Q. for all practical purposes, could identify the day and time. That is the power of Love. I learned that to express or experience Love, you do not need brains. Sheela taught me this great truth!

Transformation in Tondiarpet Home

At Tondiarpet(suburb of Chennai) home, there were nearly 400 children, most had pot belly; they wore torn clothes, had dirty teeth, smelling awful and totally unkempt. Though the campus was large for them to play, the buildings were dilapidated and not well maintained. This was a mini prison with Police sentries outside. Most of them had scabies and other skin conditions – nutrition and hygiene were totally unsatisfactory. I met the lady warden and two cooks, both ladies – who in contrast were obese. I enquired about quantity of milk given to children and was stunned by the reply. The warden said they buy eight bottles of milk (4 litres)(Those days there were no sachets). They would boil four liters of milk, make curds, and then 50 cups of buttermilk. By turn, each child would get a cup of buttermilk once a week. The food consisted of kanji(rice broth) with salt twice a day and a Sunday special with jaggery. No vegetables. I enquired about nail cutting. The warden said she herself does this. She had only one nail cutter. 20 nails x 400 children was an impossible proposition. I also found out that there was no coconut oil or hair combs available. Once in a year, a contract barber tonsured all children (boys and girls). Finally, the exasperated warden said "what else do you expect us to do with Rs.12 per month per child grant that the govt. gives?

I refused to feel defeated or dejected at the prevailing circumstances. The following Sunday, during Samithi(Sai Center) meeting, I collected 20 nail cutters from the members and took them with me on Thursday visit. I divided the children into twenty groups and chose the senior most as a leader and taught the leader how to wash the hands and do the nail cutting. I entrusted them with a nail cutter each and made them responsible for twenty children in that group.

I must give credit to Mahila group, because they came in a big way to our rescue. A group of about twenty or thirty ladies arrived on a Sunday equipped with soap, towels, coconut oil, and combs. They gave a through wash to all children and tidied them up. The result was amazing. The following Sunday all children had deworming and anti scabies treatment.

On alternate Sundays, the Mahila used to bring with them Chappathi rolling platforms and rollers and with flour and vegetables provided by the Samithi, prepare Chappathis and serve two per child along with hot vegetables. For the first time, children started eating with relish. I taught the group of children to raise kitchen garden and supplied them with tools. Soon they started consuming garden fresh vegetables. I decided not to waste the pillion seat on my scooter and each

Thursday brought a new visitor to the home. One such visitor supplied a truck load of "Bondan Valzhai"(banana) saplings and assisted in raising a huge patch of Banana plants. Mahilas used to prepare special dishes on festival occasions and feed the children. Thus nutrition was well covered. Samithi members started to donate clothes, books etc. The Secretary, Sri. G. Chunni Lal used to bring his 16 mm projector and screen cartoons once a month. Mahilas started teaching Bhajan singing. In this atmosphere, children felt embraced by the love of Sai.

The annual tonsuring practice was stopped. It was a heart warming sight to see a young girl running to me to show off her pig tails and the new ribbon provided by Mahilas.

By Swami's grace, we were able to organize a medical camp with all specialists, and pediatricians. I had invited Sri. Ra. Ganapathy, a respected author and senior devotee to preside, so that he could write about the orphanage to various journals and magazines. The skin specialist visiting the camp gave a mimicry show to entertain the children. It was a all around successful event due to Swami's grace.

As a footnote, I like to share a spiritual lesson I imbibed through this experience. The circumstances were daunting no doubt. If we are sincere and steady in our effort, Bhagawan confers His grace and ensures success. Ask and it shall be given, said Jesus. Our experience is that in Sai's work, start doing and all that is needed will be given by Him.

School Health Checkup Scheme

A special health status card was designed and printed with the Sai organization logo. Because many corporation schools could not afford to pay for doctors to conduct a check-up for all children, it was decided that Sai Organization would offer this service and give a health status report and counsel parents of children with medical problems. Being part of teaching faculty at the Madras Medical College(MMC), I was able to enlist post-graduates to volunteer for this work. During this program, two other professors from M.M.C. also joined the team – Prof. C.S. Lakshmi Narayana, Director of the P.G. Institute of Microbiology and Prof. Sharada Subramaniam of Physiology dept., and a visiting examiner for the Royal College, London. There were an enthusiastic band of young Sevadals who were eager to join this service. The Samithi secretary, Sri. G. Chunni Lal, would spare his Matador van and his driver for this Sunday service. This team of doctors and Sevadals were popularly called "Sunday Gentlemen". This service became the fore runner of SaiKrupa.

A set up team consisting of two sevadals and myself would visit the school on Saturday and set up furniture in a set pattern, put up organization banner, and ensure that logistics were in place. In this manner it was ensured that doctors' time was spent productively on Sunday.

The program schedule ran something like this: Hoisting of Prashanthi flag, bhajans for 10 minutes, followed by medical check up for children. Following registration, we'd have height and weight recorded along with relevant medical history and immunization data. This was followed by vision test, test for colour blindness, and hearing test – these tests were conducted by trained volunteers, following which doctors did a thorough clinical screening and recorded findings.

Though not common today, in those days, it wasn't unusual to see quite a few cases of 'Vitamin A' deficiency, night blindness (if untreated could lead to blindness), and chronic pus discharge from ears(leading to deafness if untreated). Suitable advice was given directly or through school authorities. Occasionaly, we'd see early stages of leprosy and suitable advice given. For cases with undescended testes, hare lip, cleft palate, enlarged tonsils and adenoids, suitable surgical intervention was adviced.

Later life morbidity and functional loss could be avoided by routine screening of children of school going age and by taking appropriate remedies. As we gained more experience and our volunteers more exposure, we were able to extend this service to orphanages, old age homes, and special homes in the city of Chennai.

As more and more volunteers joined this Sunday service, we started screening our Balvikas children and Sevadals. We included blood grouping in this screening. A special ID card for Sevadals was designed with blood group information.

From Chaos to Order and Harmony

The Sunday service became a contagious affair, and more and more young volunteers offered their services. Bhagawan says "look with eyes of compassion and an opportunity for seva will stare at you". I went around General Hospital scouting for opportunities for seva. I found that daily out patients of nearly 8000-10000 find it difficult to join the long queues. There was a crying need for volunteers to regulate and guide the vast numbers to the right dept. About 15 Sevadals agreed to spare two hours from 7.00 a.m. to 9.00 a.m. Soon the confusion and chaos of the outpatient dept. was resolved and the courteous and ever smiling volunteers with scarf were in great demand by the R.M.O(Resident Medical Officer) as well as O.P. Doctors. Such was impact of "Sai Seva". This service continued for many years and formed a training ground for the future SaiKrupa Volunteers. Veerabadriah, a senior sevadal who has been a member of the medical team for almost 4 decades had this to say:

"General Hospital duty was a great learning experience, especially in crowd management and maintaining harmony and order. For example, there used to be different queues for B-Complex and Antibiotics in the Injection O.P. Dept. Very often, after having stood for more than an hour outside they used to discover that they are in the wrong line and had to join a second line and wait another hour. This used to lead to a lot of heart burn and quarreling. We used to quickly check the O.P. tickets and guide them to proper lines.

Nearly 30% of patients used to walk in from Central Railway Station, having arrived there from Andhra Pradesh. Some could talk Tamil but very few could read Tamil & English boards. Their confused faces would say it all. By speaking Telugu I would put them at ease and assist them to their satisfaction. Having picked up a smattering of Hindi also, I was in great demand by O.P. doctors."

Sri. Venkatraghavan – the senior most of Saidapet brothers is vociferous in telling that "the General Hospital service gave us a good grounding in managing patients. A ready smile, a helping hand, an offer of drinking water or a wheel chair made us very popular with the patients. I think wearing a scarf(pink in those days) sort of created a status of authority and our manners made strangers seek help from us. On the days when regular staff were either late or absent, the R.M.O. would utilize our services for issuing O.P. tickets, manning registers, and even pharmacy counters for packing tablets, labeling mixture bottles and dispensing ointments. We were sort of multipurpose utilities used as a solution to any problem. Soon the chaos that was

General Hospital O.P. settled down to smooth running well greased machinery. In the bargain, we were blessed to acquire new skills while offering Sai Seva."

Sri. Gopalakrishnan – our sevadal leader – is all smiles while recounting his General Hospital days. "In the surgical O.P. we learnt the requirement of surgeons and the order in which they are to be handed. At the surgeon's nod with his eye movement to one of us, we would take the patient behind the screens, undress, make them lie down on the couch and be ready for a detailed internal examination. The nurses used to marvel at how quickly we learnt to handle sterile things and asisst the doctor with gloves and implements. The surgeons were happiest at the professional way in which we learnt to help them out."

As a corollary I would like to mention this incident.

In our operating theatre we had a changing room with lockers etc. where we used to order and have coffee and snacks in between sessions of surgery. All my friends knew that on Thursdays I would have only coffee and not snacks. One of the surgical PG's was inquisitive to know which Baba I followed – the old man or the hippie with African hair –do? My answer was in the form of a query: whether he has seen the volunteers with scarf in the O.P.? He was awestruck and said "If that is the tail end of your Sai organization, I can imagine what the head must be .Hats off to your Baba."

"To improve and maintain the health of the people, continuous education on the principles and practice of hygiene, and environmental cleanliness is essential. Education is more effective safeguard against physical and mental ill health" – Baba, Aug 28th, 1976

Blood Donation Campaign

In General Hospital, Madras, during the mid 70's, surgery was frequently postponed for want of blood. There were very few voluntary donors. General awareness of blood donation was not there. Professional donors used to demand a huge price especially during emergency surgery requiring urgent blood transfusion. Hence it was decided to start a blood donation campaign. A set of slides was prepared to raise awareness amongst devotees about blood donation as a service. Soon thereafter, a mini blood donation camp was organized at Abbottsbury. The devotees who were singing bhajans would go, offer blood and come back and resume singing. This was a great motivator and removed the lurking fear in the minds of other devotees who were singing. The idea-that you donate blood in this atmosphere…blood has the additional benefit of your prayer and doubly benefits the patient - caught on. There were no dearth of volunteers and SaiKrupa blood donation camps became very popular. For the annual World Blood Donation Day, Sai Organization was awarded 'Maximum Donors Prize' for several years.

Annual Global Blood Donation was conducted at Abbotsbury as the hall was available. The dining hall was converted into a ward with ten couches on either side along with side tables and chair for the person collecting blood. Such a big facility was nonexistent even in big teaching hospitals with transfusion medicine as a special subject.

We worked with city hospitals and Red Cross - they came with equipment, Nurses and ancillary staff to collect blood. On average, 200 to 250 voluntary donors from Sai organization were present. The physical checkup was conducted by Saikrupa team, the organization provided infrastructure and refreshments to the donor. Once Abbotsbury was no longer available, this service was done at two or three teaching hospitals simultaneously.

We have witnessed the progress of tools and technology: from blood bottles and autoclaved red and green rubber blood sets to the disposable vacuum sachets with disposable polyethylene blood sets.

During Bhagawan's 60th birthday, the American Red Cross had issued a certificate in the name of "Sri Sathya Sai Baba" for motivating a large number of donors(published in Beacon) and from then on this service was referred as "liquid love".

Blood donation had become a sought after service opportunity that on one occasion we had hard time convincing an old lady donor that because of age and low hemoglobin she wouldn't be able to donate. Her plea was that we should take atleast half bottle of blood and give to a child or a baby. It was inspiring for all of us to experience her sense of devotion.

When Bhagawan was informed that there were more women volunteers offering blood, He had a word of praise for their sense of sacrifice: "men can hardly match them", He said.

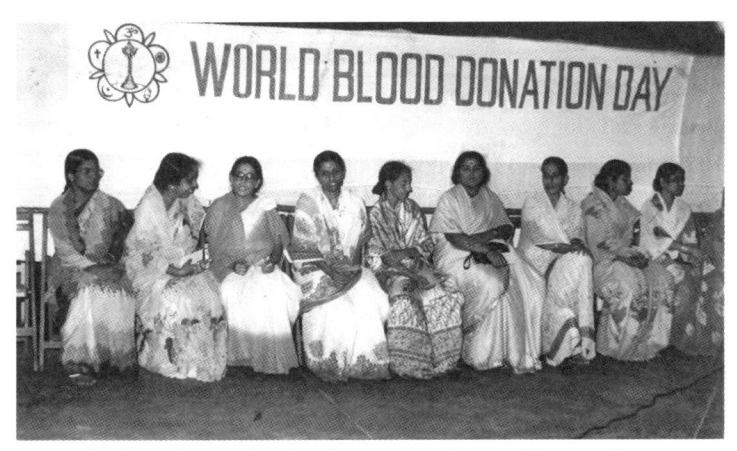

Ladies in the Sai Organization have come forward in amazing numbers to take part in blood donation. It is little wonder that their service touched Swami's heart and elicited a word of praise.

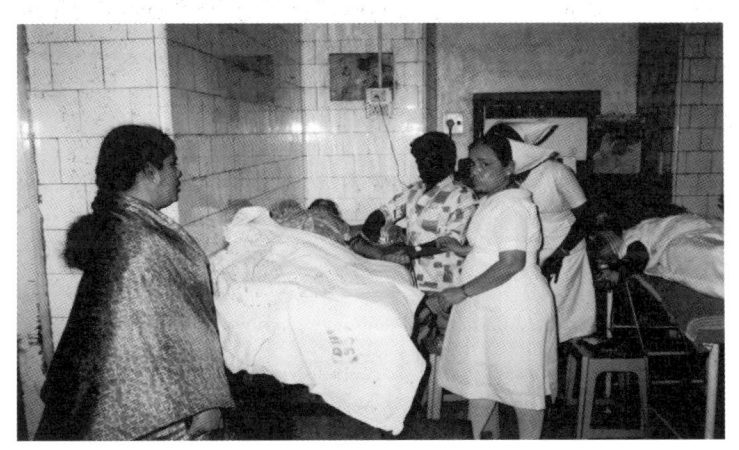

Technician prepares a lady volunteer for blood donation

24x7 Blood Donation Service at Sundaram

A team of volunteers led by Sri. Thyagarajan started propagating the benefits of Liquid Love donation at various schools and other Institutions with a missionary zeal. Sri. Thyagarajan with the aid of a computer started maintaining donors' data and started responding to emergency calls. This Liquid Love service got a permanent home at Sundaram with a special cubical, a computer, a telephone line and 24x7 volunteer service from 1998. This service round the clock responded to the emergency calls from the hospitals for a particular group of blood. From the data available, they would ring up the nearest donor available and depute him/her to the concerned hospital or nursing home. This service, which is only one of a kind in the city, is very popular. In addition, announcements were also made after bhajans on Thursdays and Sundays at Sundaram for planned cardiac and other major surgeries requiring more than one donor. This was continued for 15 years. As calls for the night service became less and less, currently this service is restricted to hours of 9:00 a.m. to 8:00 p.m.

Long after Sri. Thygarajan handed over this service to Sundaram and was assigned bigger responsibilities, he continues to be affectionately referred as "liquid love" Thygarajan. Tens of thousands of patients have benefitted since inception of this service.

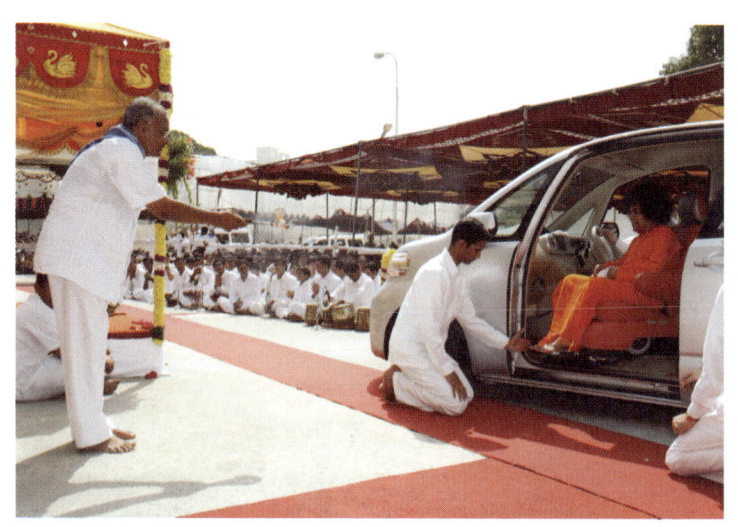

Liquid Love Thyagarajan offering Aarati to the
Ocean of Love – Sundaram, Jan. 2007

Relay Medical Service – Story of Joseph

Extending medical service to rural patients requiring specialized treatment available only at Madras - in those days - was a topic of frequent discussion. The opportunity and the means to deliver this service to a rural patient materialized in a miraculous way.

Joseph was a robust young man of 19 years working as a painter for a building contractor. He was an orphan who was brought up by this contractor from his young age. He had learnt the art of painting rafters, doors and windows, etc. One fine morning he found that he could not climb the ladder to reach the rafter in the ceiling. There was weakness in his legs. The next day he developed weakness in his arms and could not even lift a brush. He was admitted in the Coimbatore Headquarters Hospital. The doctors diagnosed a problem in the spinal cord, recommended urgent surgery, and advised him to be shifted to Madras. Unable to move all the four limbs, Jospeh was totally helpless and bed ridden. The contractor was willing to pay for the treatment but could not mobilize two volunteers to take him to Madras and stay with him until the treatment was completed. It was a sad situation. On discharge, Joseph was taken to "Nirmal Hruday" - A Home for dying destitutes, run by Mother Theresa.

Dr. Punnaivanam who was a visiting doctor to Nirmal Hruday saw Joseph within a few hours of his admission there. Same night, he called and enquired whether something can be done for this patient at Madras. I promised to make enquiries with the Neurosurgery department and get back to him. The following morning, even before I could enquire at the Neurosurgery department, I received a phone message from home stating that Dr. Punnaivanam had dispatched the patient along with two Sevadals wearing scarves by West Coast Express. I was requested to receive the patient at Central Station by 12:30 p.m. that day. I was shocked since there was no way to leave the operation theatre where I was working, before 2:00 p.m. that day. I made frantic phone calls to Sri. Chunni Lal, the Samithi secretary, requesting him to take his van to the Central Station, receive the patient and wait there till I could free myself and reach Central Station. Strangely, surgery scheduled for 12:00 p.m. was cancelled for want of blood... I could rush to Central Station by 12:30 p.m. just as the West Coast Express was moving into Platform #1. I could identify the volunteers with the scarves and shifted the patient into the van brought by the secretary and drove down to General Hospital which is opposite to the Central Station. Joseph was admitted to Neuro Ward. The elevator which was under repair for nearly a couple of months had been repaired and was ready for service. What would have been a difficult and long journey for the patient to reach the sixth floor was made very easy. A bed that had just fallen vacant was offered for this patient – it is very rare for a patient to walk-in and be assigned a bed. I re-assured the patient that everything would be alright and that I would talk to the surgeon next morning and left.

The following morning, after settling routine work in operation theatre, I went to meet Dr. V. Balasubramaniam in order to request him to operate on Joseph at an early date. When I reached the Neuro Theatre, I found Dr. V. Balasubramaniam removing his mask and coming out. He started off saying "Dr. Vijai Kumar, don't you know Spinal Cord compression is a surgical emergency. You should have called me last night itself. Anyway, don't worry I have completed the surgery just now. He had a congenital band and I have removed the same. He will be alright." I was stunned. I had come to request early surgery only to find that the patient was already operated.

Joseph stayed in the hospital for six weeks for physiotherapy, picked up good friendship with the Sevadals who were visiting him daily and because of their company he gave up smoking. When he was discharged he could walk back to Central Station (with the help of a walking stick) and return to Coimbatore. Joseph was a new man looking forward to a new life – a man who was an orphan and who was admitted to a home for dying destitutes. Who made all this happen? Bhagawan's ways are mysterious. He is the doer. Occasionally, He parts the curtain and allows us to see who's behind the scene and makes us aware of our role in His drama.

Under the relay medical service another patient was referred from Erode and was able to get an artificial limb fitted at General Hospital, Madras.

> "It is your good fortune that you have become doctors. Sacrifice is the hall mark of a true doctor. So, doctors should have a spirit of sacrifice. They should be compassionate and considerate towards the poor. There are many poor people who are loosing their lives as they cannot afford costly treatment. Your love alone can sustain such lives. The more you develop the spirit of sacrifice in you, the greater will be world's progress." – Baba, Jan 19, 2001

Sai Supports

Swami says that one only needs to see with eyes of compassion to find an opportunity to serve. Sevadals visiting General Hospital spotted an opportunity to serve. They witnessed a number of accident cases and many patients who had lost their legs could not be rehabilitated with crutches. There was no provision to buy and supply crutches for deserving patients. They did not have any budget for it. Sevadals decided to do something about it and went about it seriously. They were able to locate a timber merchant who was a devotee - he not only was willing to provide the Wood free of cost but also offer the services of his carpenter free of cost. Another devotee who was a hardware merchant came forward to offer bolts and nuts. The only item on which they had to pay cash was for the foam cushion. Thus the manufacture of crutches, which they named as "Sai – Supports", was started. General Hospital used to refer amputees to "SaiKrupa" for providing crutches. This service went on for several years until the Government sanctioned a budget for this item. By Swami's grace, this service still continues at SaiKrupa. Now not only Sai – Supports but also walking sticks for the blind with a spring bell made of Aluminum are provided free of cost to the patients. Sai Supports have themselves improved from wood to aluminum and with rubber shoes and better cushions. Many Sai families sponsor the manufacturing costs as a way of celebrating family member's birthdays as well as other ceremonies.

I must narrate the transformative impact of Sai Supports. Murugan was admitted to Anna Cancer Hospital, Kancheepuram, for a swelling in his thigh. He was hardly 22 years old, had been newly married and with a baby 3 months old. On investigation it was found that he had Cancer of his thigh bone. His affected leg had to be amputated at the hip level. The doctors told him that his life expectancy was 6 months to a maximum of 1 year. Murugan was so depressed that he refused to talk to anybody or even play with his own baby. He had lost all interest in life. I happened to be working at this hospital during that time and I carried with me a pair of Sai Supports from Madras to Kanchipuram by bus and taught Murugan how to use the Sai Supports. This made all the difference. Murugan wanted to be discharged immediately. His plea was "I have only one year left, I would like to go and work somewhere so that I can leave some money for my wife and child". A depressed person got back his self – confidence -that is SaiKrupa.

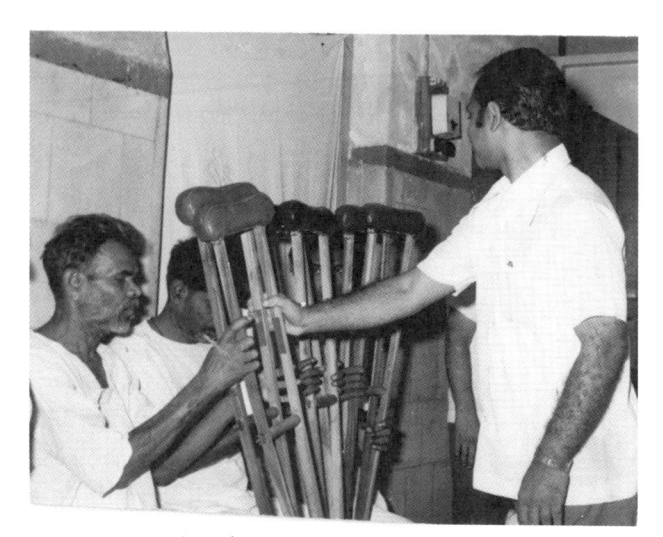

A patient receiving Sai Supports

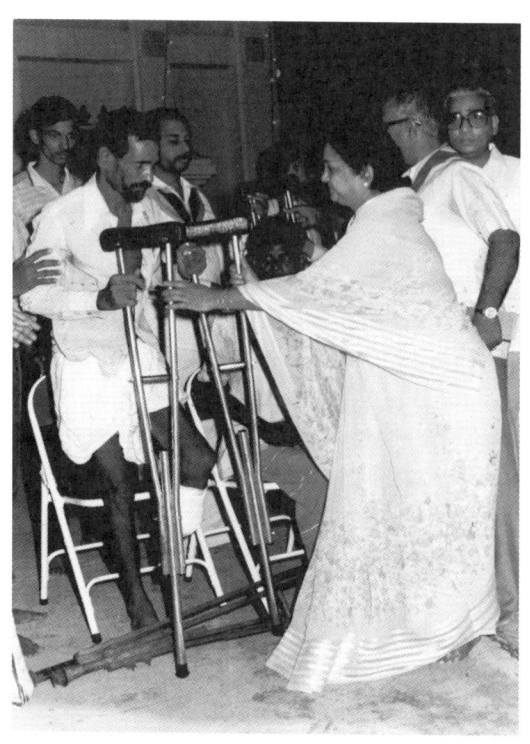

Patient receives Sai Supports from
Smt. Anjali Devi, an ardent devotee of Bhagawan

Hands that Help are Holier than Lips that Pray

As the School Health Check – up Program and Orphanage service were becoming more popular more doctors specially devotee doctors started volunteering for service. Earliest to join were three sisters from the same family of Bhagawan's devotees. They had started as sevadal volunteers and later qualified as doctors and joined the team. They were Dr. Rama Devi, Dr. Lakshmi Devi, and Dr. Girija Devi – the first two being twins. Dr. Kumari Menon also started attending along with Prof. Sharada Subramaniam. Dr. G. V. Ramakrishnan who was appointed by Bhagawan Himself as a member of Madras Samithi in 1967 also joined the team. Dr. A. Sudhakar Rao followed him after a few months.

I was encouraged by then President of Madras Samithi, Sri. T.G. Krishnamurthy, to organize an exhibition on seva activities. By Swami's grace, I had a good collection of photographs of Swami and Service activities. Several artists worked to get a professional quality exhibition ready in a months' time. All boards had to be designed, painted and lettering had to be done by hand brush (there were no computers or printers available at that time). The title was Bhagawan's words - "Hands that Help are Holier than the Lips that Pray". The display also included two large panels on blood donation and eye donation. This first ever exhibition at Abbottsbury was inaugurated by Sri. Patwari, then Governor of Tamil Nadu.

An improved version was also subsequently exhibited at Rajeshwari Kalyana Mandapam during Bhagawan's visit. Swami went around and looked at each exhibit in detail along with a batch of students who had accompanied Him. This experience laid the foundation and I was blessed to organize exhibitions several times including the Indian Section of the International Medical Exhibition during the conference at Prashanthi Nilayam in the year 2005.

> "Doctors should infuse courage in patients and speak soothingly, radiating compassion and love. While your are examining a patient, you should have a smiling face and talk to the patient sweetly."– Baba, Feb 6, 1993

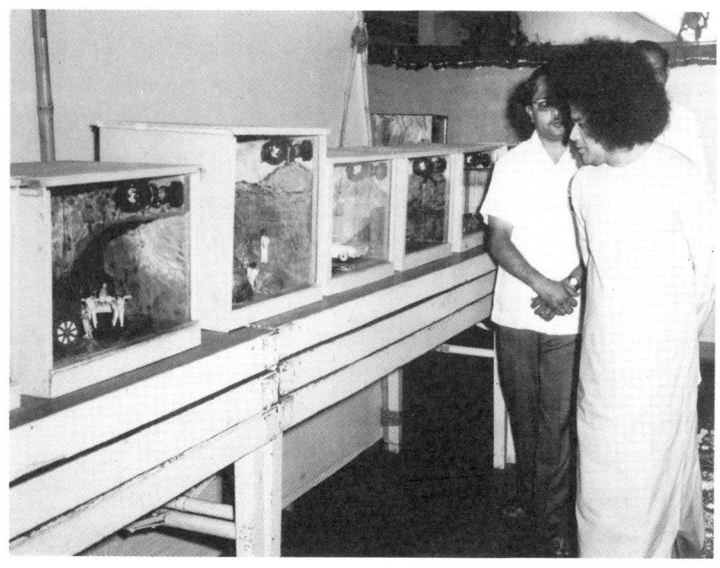

Bhagawan visiting Exhibits in Rajeswari Kalyana Mandapam

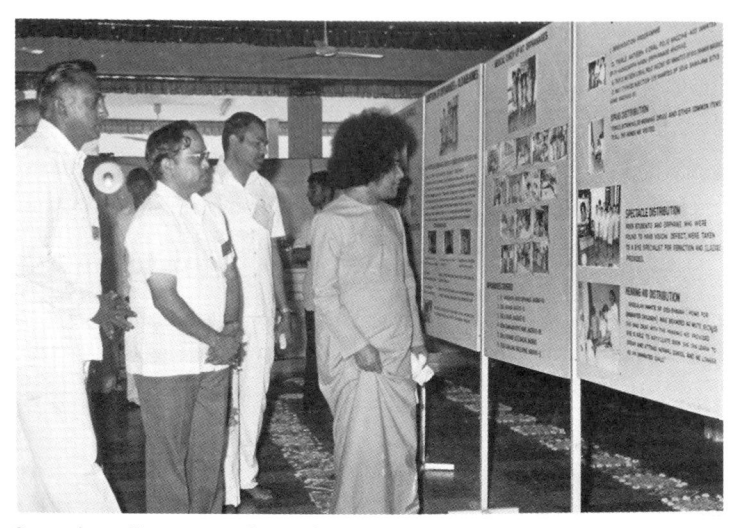

Swami reading story of transformation at the orphanage in Tondiarpet

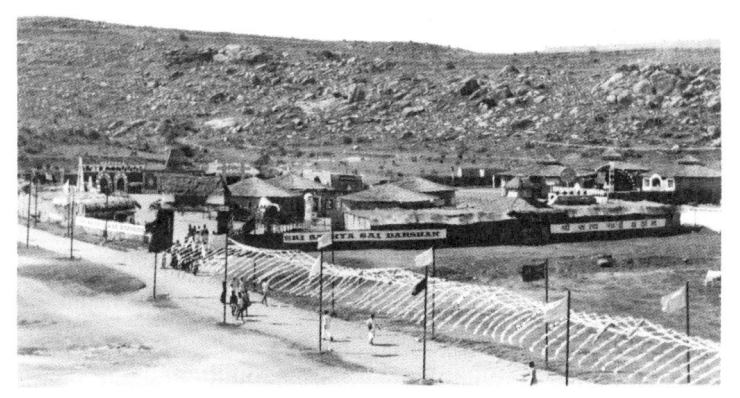

'Sri Sathya Sai Darshan'- Exhibition during 60th birthday, 1984, at Hill view Stadium, Puttaparthi

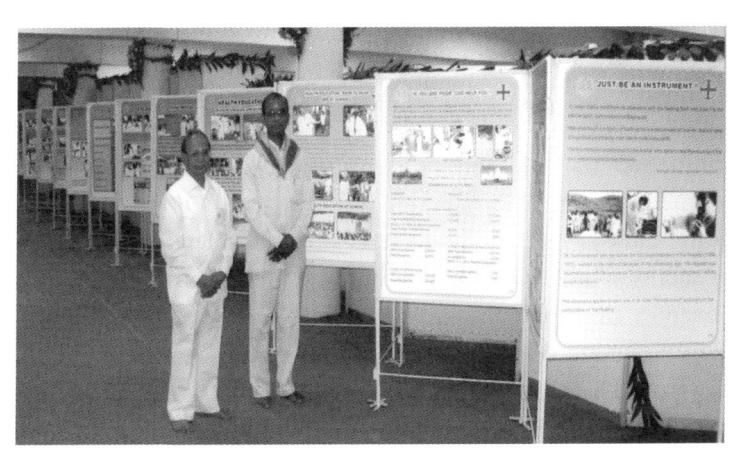

Indian section of International Medical Exhibition at Double Decker Building, Puttaparthi, 2005

Sai Free Clinics in the City

As the medical man power increased and the work force of sevadal grew, the idea of permanent weekly clinics was mooted. Mrs. Radha Menon of Kilpauk came forward with the offer of an out-house in her backyard for this purpose. Bhagawan graciously inaugurated this clinic on 15th January 1978. Bhagawan blessed all the doctors, lighted the lamp and signed in OP register. He also visited the main residential portion and blessed the members of the family of "Radhamma" as Bhagawan used to call her. She was in – charge of Sai Bala Gurukulam at Sai Nivas, Perambur.

The very same evening, Bhagawan inaugurated another free clinic at Mandaveli (Suburb of Chennai) in Dr. Narayan Rao's house. Dr. Sharadha Subramaniam and myself who had opted to serve in the clinic, were fortunate to be blessed by Bhagawan at this time. Dr. Sharadha Subramaniam also started another free clinic in her garage at Nungambakkam – a suburb of Chennai. The Kilpauk clinic was functioning on Sunday mornings and the Mandaveli and Nungambakkam clinics were functioning on Thursday afternoons. On Sundays, I could take turns with other Doctors but on Thursdays, I had to divide my time between duty at General Hospital, visit to orphanages, and the Sai Clinics. In due course of time, two sevadals graduated from Medical College to become Doctors - they were Dr. C. Rajkumar from Madras Medical College and Dr. Shiva Subramaniam from Stanley Medical College.

Healthcare has been extensively studied by economists. Who pays for healthcare and how to make healthcare universally available and economically viable? This is a question facing every country. USA has a mix of private and govt. Funded healthcare. United Kindgom's healthcare bill is paid in large part by the govt. In India, majority of healthcare is borne by private citizens, govt. share of the pie is a small fraction. The United Nations and World Health Organization has a massive budget for healthcare. I cannot help being awestruck at the simple & effective ways in which Swami helped us set up healthcare for the needy in Chennai. We didn't start with a budget, we started with a prayer and a yearning to serve - Swami backed us with necessary resources. People came forward to offer their space, skills, and everything we required started to fall in place. To start good works, money is not a pre-requisite, as much as purity of purpose and selflessness. Money and resources necessarily follow good & noble deeds and not the other way around. This is the lesson we experienced.

Here, I want to add a word to the young and the young-at-heart who are driven to do noble deeds of service. Sai Organization offers us a platform to do noble deeds without the usual constraints of fund raising that is at the heart of many organizations. This is the uniqueness of Sai Organization. Goddess of wealth – Lakshmi – follows her Lord Narayana where ever He may go. Here, Lord Narayana is symbolic of noble deeds. Wealth of resources - of men and material and skills necessarily follows good deeds. Sai Organization the world over stands as a shining example for this principle of service to needy at its core as opposed to fund raising.

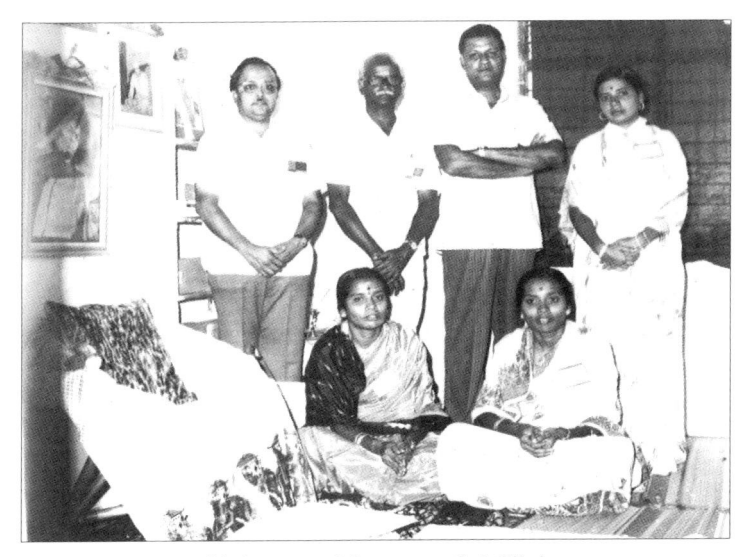

Initial group of doctors at Sai Clinics

Standing(L to R) Dr. M. Vijai Kumar, Dr. G. V. Ramakrishna,
Dr. A. Sudhakar Rao, Dr. Girija Devi. Sitting(L to R)
Dr. Rama Devi, Dr. Lakshmi Devi

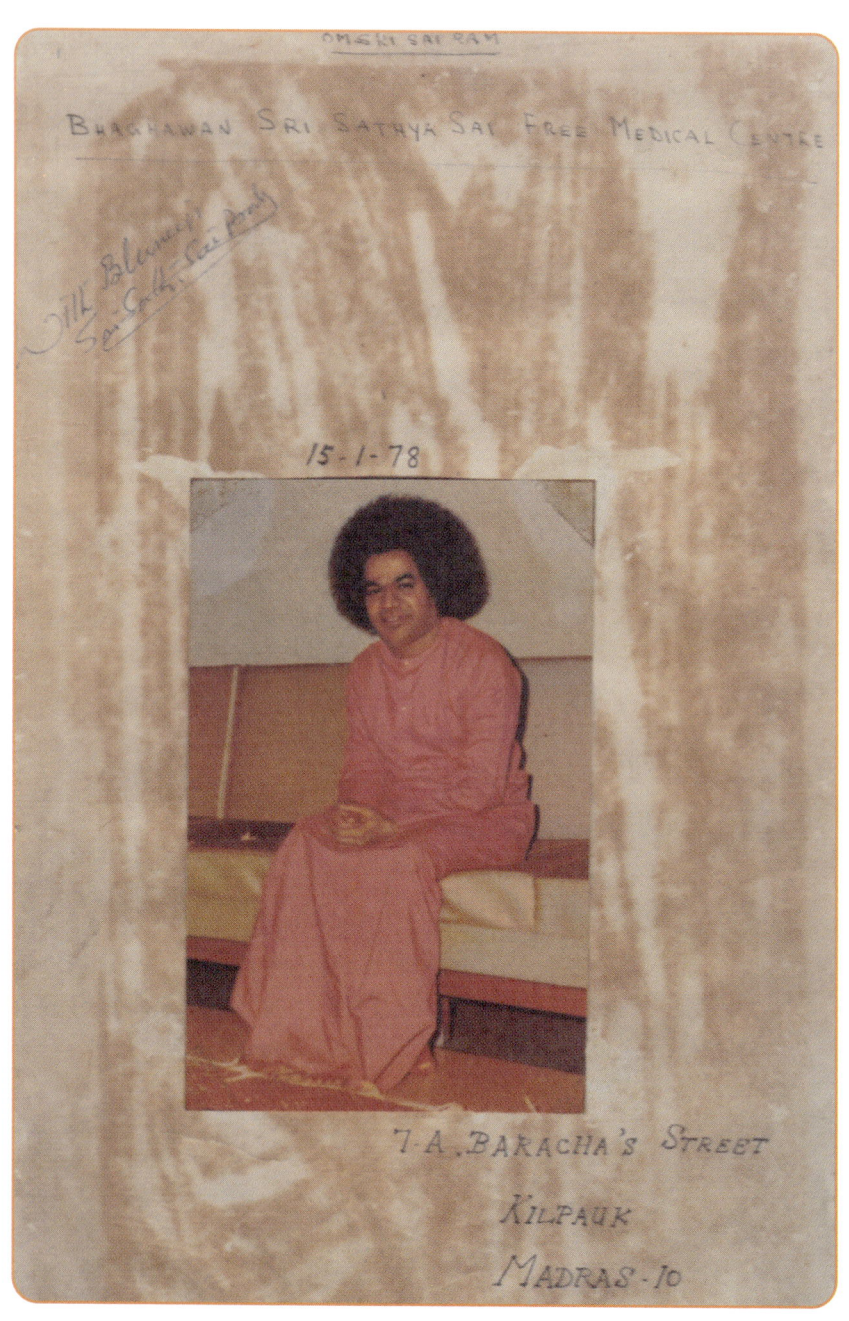

First page of Patient Register at inauguration of
Kilpauk Sai Clinic was blessed with Bhagawan's autograph

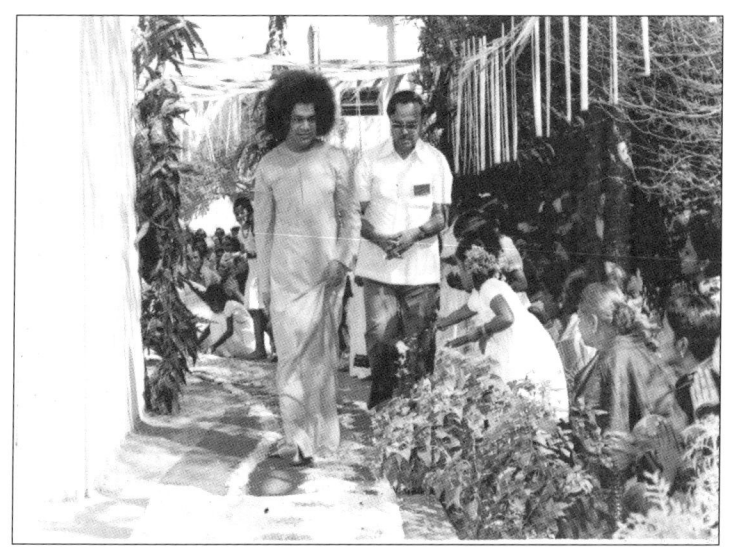

Bhagawan arrives to bless Kilpauk Sai Clinic – Jan. 15, 1978

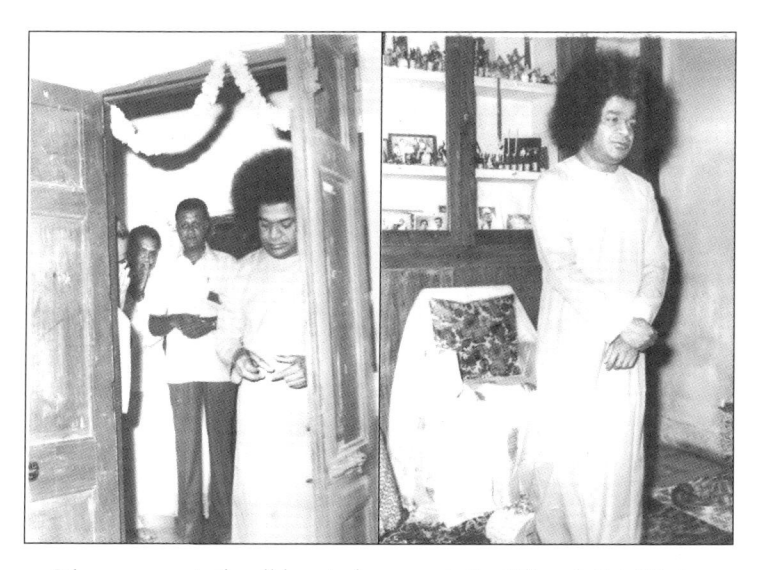

Bhagawan cuts the ribbon to inaugurate the Kilpauk Sai Clinic.
With a simple movement of scissor's arm,
Bhagawan cuts the tie between a patient and misery.
Seen behind Bhagawan – Sri. N. Ramani and Dr. A. Sudhakar Rao

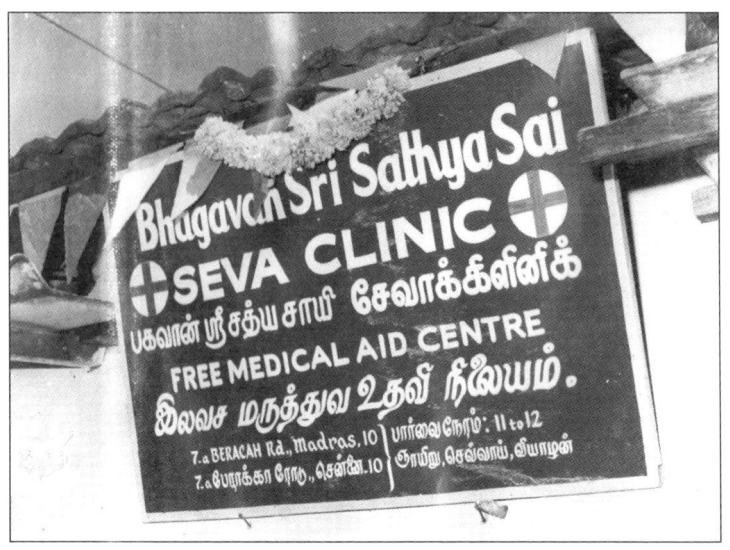

A simple black board at entrance to Sai Clinic at Kilpauk.
OP hours: 11 – 12 on Tue, Thu, Sun.

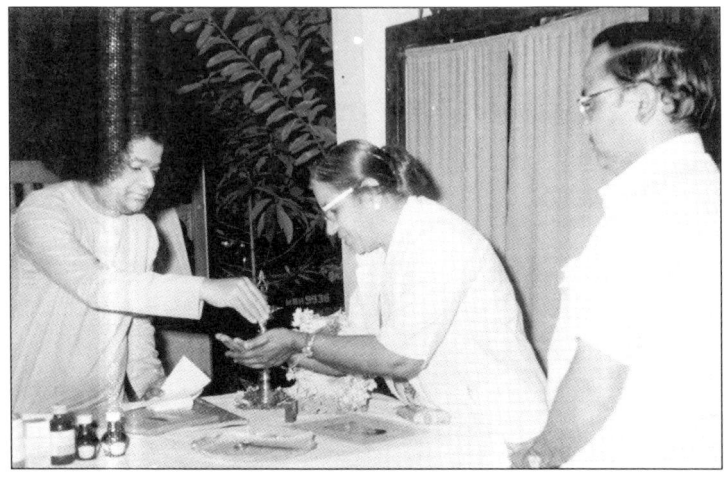

Bhagawan blessing Dr. Sharada Subramanium and Dr. M. Vijai Kumar after inaugurating Sai Clinic in Mandaveli, Jan. 15, 1978

Birth of SaiKrupa

Bhagawan's modus operandi - if I could call it so - has often been low key and high impact. All His epoch making works were announced without fanfare, often times in the most non-chalant manner, as a casual matter-of-fact in the midst of His discourse. For the One who prompts words, no press conference in necessary – every act of His is the subject of spiritual conferences for time to come.

The birth of SaiKrupa bore similar evidence of being a divine progeny. Events colluded, as it were, to usher SaiKrupa to the world. The state government of Tamil Nadu of which Chennai is the capital had promulgated the Urban Land Ceiling Act. Because of this, there was a chance of losing a patch of open parking space in the Abbottsbury compound(Wedding Hall owned by Sathya Sai Trust). Swami sent word that the space should be utilized for a free medical center. This was during the end of April 1979. The trust got ready with a thatched structure 30'x60' within a weeks time and on Easwaramma Day, 6th May 1979 "SAIKRUPA" was inaugurated by Sri. Manickyavachagam, then State President of Tamil Nadu Sai Organisation.

Few chairs and tables could be borrowed from Abbottsbury itself. I brought my BP apparatus and stethoscope with a box of sample medicines and the work got started off. Because there was no time for planning or publicity, I had requested the watchman at the gate to be the first patient, promising him a big tonic bottle. The word got around and on the day of inauguration, a few doctors could serve nearly 50 patients.

Within a short time, SaiKrupa became well known, patients from far off places started seeking treatment. Within a year, we had nearly 100 doctors on our panel, serving about 900 – 1000 patients at this Sunday outpatient service, every week. Dr. V. K. Gokak, Vice Chancellor of Sri Sathya Sai Insititute of Higher Learning happened to visit SaiKrupa and was stunned at the silent Sai Seva. He sought and published an article on SaiKrupa in Sai Chandana -the very first publication of the Sai University.

Homeopathy Clinic

In less than a year of starting Sai Krupa, Dr. Easwaran – a Homeopathy practitioner joined the team. We had a separate section serving those patients seeking Homeopathy treatment. Dr. Easwaran trained a band of committed lady volunteers to do the intricate homeopathy dispensing. He was a much respected colleague at

SaiKrupa and served along with us for more than 3 decades until his passing 2 years ago. His assistants and his daughter who is also qualified, staff the homeopathy section currently.

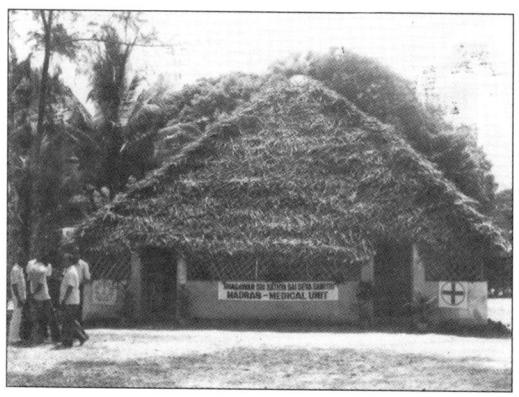

SaiKrupa was housed in a thatched roof building, in the campus of Abbotsbury wedding hall, Chennai, in 1979. Inner motivation draws Lord's compassion and grace than the parade of outer accoutrements

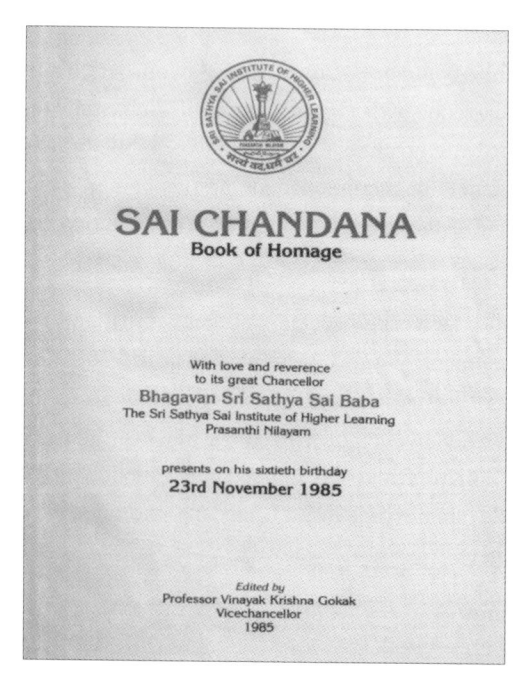

Dr. V.K. Gokak published an article on SaiKrupa in Sai Chandana – very first publication of Sri Sathya Sai Institute of Higher Learning

Medicine Bank

The word of mouth publicity created awareness of SaiKrupa and it experienced a steady increase in the number of patients seeking and receiving treatment. Medicines procured by Doctors with their meager budget for a month, used to be exhausted within two weeks. I was working in Government General Hospital at that time, where it was a practice for medical representatives(reps) to meet doctors during lunch hour at the DAS Quarters (Duty Assistant Surgeons Quarters) and offer promotional literature and sample medicines. Popular practitioners would attract large supplies of these medicines. I used to go around meeting these reps and tell them about SaiKrupa and collect samples. After a few days, they themselves offered to collect the samples among themselves in a big box and deliver the same at SaiKrupa. Sri. N. Ramani - then sevadal leader(currently National Vice President) - was himself from Pharmaceutical industry and had volunteered to work in SaiKrupa dispensary. Sri. N. Ramani used to liaise with other suppliers and mobilize large quantities of "Medicine Contribution" for SaiKrupa Medicine Bank.

Sri. Viswanathan of LIC, three Saidapet brothers who were dedicated Sai Sevaks, Sri. Balan, Sri. Manoharan of Perambur were a great team of workers who would go around and collect sample medicines from doctors' clinics. They used to form a "sorting team" under the leadership of Dr. C. Rajkumar to classify and put the medicines in various boxes, and label them as Antibiotic, Anti – Emetics and Anti – Diarrhea, etc. so that they could be dispensed easily. "Soiled Carton" boxes also used to form a major source. If one bottle was broken, entire carton was discarded. We used to leverage unbroken bottle of medicines that were good for us. It was decided that no injections except for emergency will be administered at SaiKrupa.

Because the work load and time constraint patients from Mandaveli and Nungambakkam were asked to attend SaiKrupa on Sundays.

The Kilpauk Dispensary still functions and is kept open. The number of patients seeking treatment here became less and less as the slum surrounding the area was replaced by multiple residential flats, and the opening of few other free dispensaries. Few chronic asthmatic patients still visit the dispensary. Radhamma helps them to procure medicines. She also does wound dressings and counseling services. All of them are particular in collecting Vibhuthi Prasadam. Sri. Mohan Ramachandran, a sevadal member, who has been offering services at the Kilpauk clinic from day 1 does not miss his Sunday service even today.

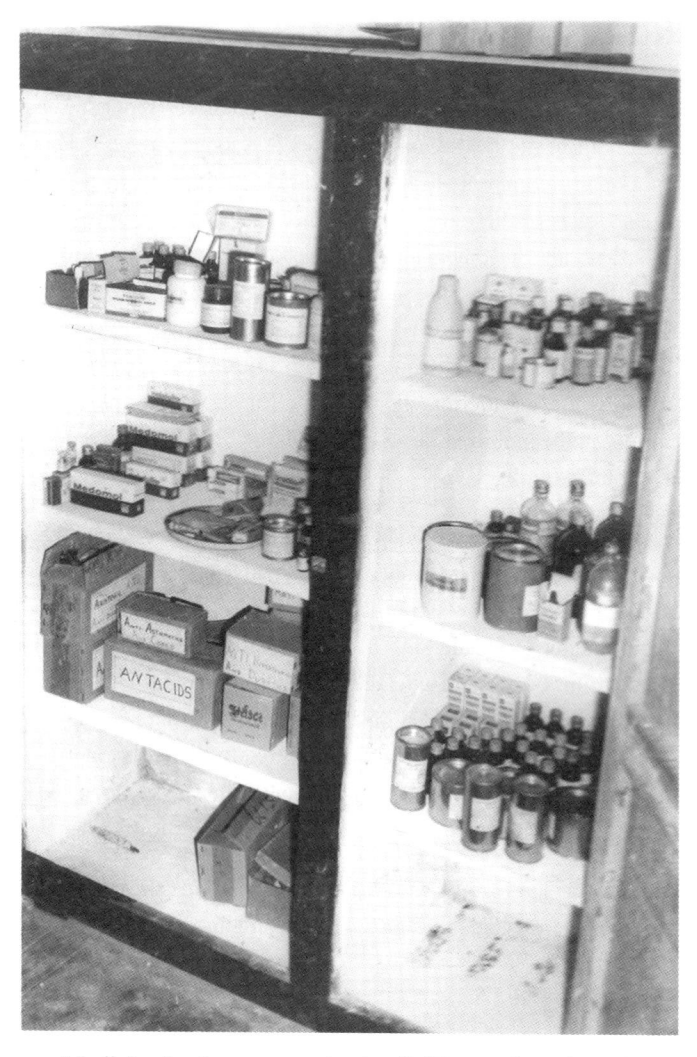

Medicine bank was organized at SaiKrupa. Sample and donated medicines were sorted in to various categories and stored for dispensing to patients

Sookshma Sai Clinical Lab

After functioning for a few Sundays with this basic facilities, we were wondering if only there was a small lab which can carry out urine tests and simple blood test, diagnoses of the condition of the patients could be clinched and better treatment could be offered. That evening, I went to Sundaram for Bhajan and wanted to request support from the Samithi Members. On reaching Sundaram, I was called in by Sri. Achuthanandam to inspect a big box received from Trichy and see if some of the contents could be utilized for SaiKrupa. I was amazed to find an imported microscope, pipettes and all ancillary equipment for establishing a clinical lab in good condition. The box had been received 4 days prior and was lying there ready to be opened. Bhagawan made the equipment available even before planting an idea for a lab in our mind. Prof. C. S. Lakshminarayana took charge of the equipment and started the lab work the very next Sunday. Proposal to name the lab as Sookshma Sai Lab was approved and blessed by Bhagawan.

Sri. Chunni Lal could organize few benches and cupboards from his factory. He started supplying tablet covers specially made in his Damodar Envelope Factory. Even today, long after his passing, and dismantling of the factory, his son Sri. Santh Kumar supplies our monthly tablet cover requirement. Sri. N. Ramani arranged to equip the dispensing section with racks, trays, boxes, jars, bottles, etc. Dr. Balaram used to supply butter milk to all doctors and volunteers. This is continued by his family even today, long after his passing. This is the bond of love built by Bhagawan. Sri. T. G. Krishnamurthy who was then district president used to visit SaiKrupa every Sunday and encourage doctors and volunteers. His support was a main stay and continued for several years inspite of his other responsibilities in Sai Organization and his frequent International tours and travels.

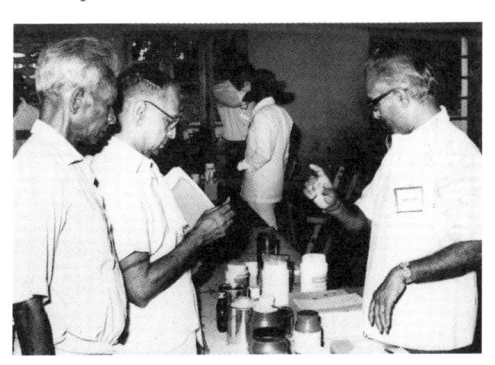

Sri.Viswanathan(Sevadal) seen dispensing medicines to patients at SaiKrupa

Sai Niketan

There were many visually challenged students in Madras...they heard about SaiKrupa and started seeking medical relief. They were very happy at the loving manner in which they were treated by the Sevadals. In those days, these students used to get free bus passes and Abbottsbury itself was a famous bus stop. For them, commuting was easy. On the request of one of them, tuition classes were started. Their main handicap was that text books in braille were not available; in addition, it was hard to find a reader who'd read the normal books such that they could take notes in braille. The big campus with a lot of shady trees and adequate folding chairs became a infrastructure for "Reading for the Blind" Service. There were many M.Com. and M.A. graduates who would volunteer their time on Sunday morning during SaiKrupa working hours. They not only read the text books but also tutored these under graduate students. There were easily 20-30 visually challenged students on any given Sunday availing this service. The volunteers also enrolled themselves in the "Readers and Writers Association" so that they would write the answer sheets on dictation by these challenged students. The amazing Sai grace was evident when they found the average pass rate of these students increase from 30% to 60% annually.

The entire atmosphere in and around SaiKrupa was suffused with love and people started to compare it with Tagore's Shanthi Niketan – a veritable SAI NIKETAN.

These challenged students were so overwhelmed by the loving atmosphere that they also wanted to join the seva activities. A couple of them transcribed in braille, Sathyam Sivam Sundaram, and were blessed to present the same directly to Bhagawan. They were also blessed to visit Prashanthi Nilayam.

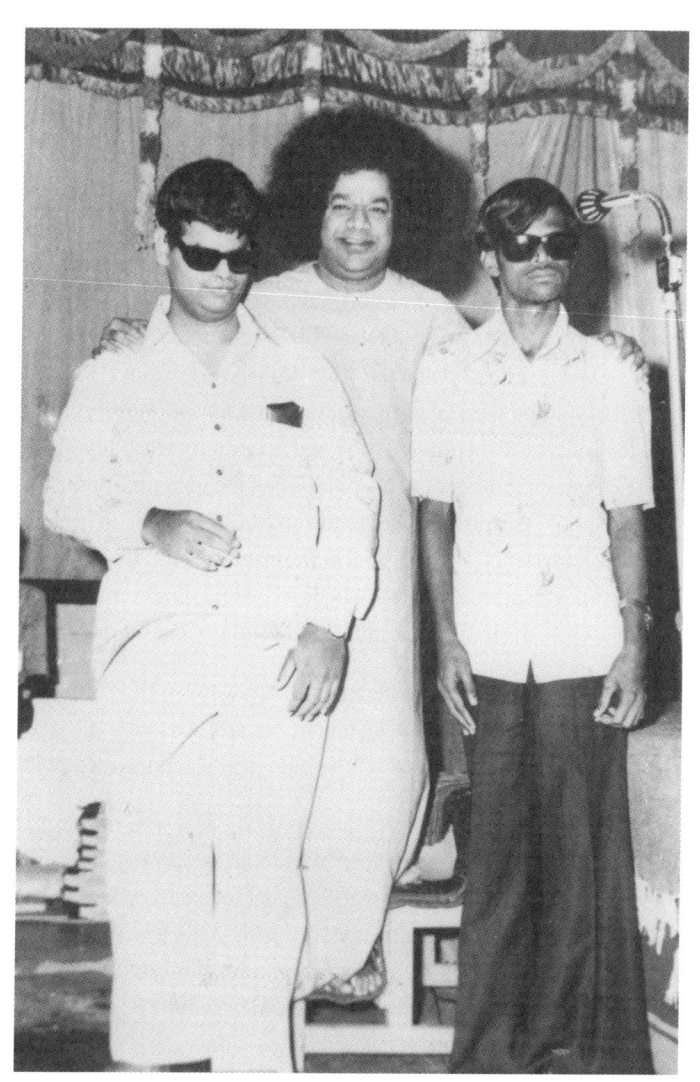

Sri. Sridhar (Swami's right) and Sri. Sriram were frequent visitors to SaiKrupa. They were inspired to transcribe Sathyam Sivam Sundaram in Braille – thereby sharing the nectarine story of Avatar of the age with visually challenged. Just as Lord Rama caressed and showered His love on the little squirrel that helped in building the bridge, Bhagawan Sri Sathya Sai baba showered His love and blessings in plenty on these students who helped spread His message. This isn't just a tale of two Avatars who appeared at different times on Earth. It is the same God, showering the same supreme love and compassion. Time is just a witness.

Sathya Sai Mission Hospital – Coimbatore

One summer during early 70's, Bhagawan was due to visit Ooty to inspect a property acquired by the Trust (in Nandanavanam). Dr. Punnaivanam was driving up to Ooty for Bhagawan's darshan - I happened to be at Coimbatore on that day and got a chance to accompany Dr. Punnaivanam. During this drive, Dr. Punnaivanam mentioned about an offer of a patch of 14 acres of land in the periphery of the city(Coimbatore), free of cost, if a free hospital is built on this site. I was excited and we began discussing the idea of a Sai Hospital. By chance, we met a devotee from USA the very next day who said that the "Salvation Army" from US with which he was connected would be interested in sending doctors and nurse volunteers who would work free of cost if accommodation and hospitality was looked after. There was also offer of equipments for the hospital. Thus the idea for building a "Sathya Sai Mission Hospital" germinated. On return to Madras, I met an architect friend and utilizing my experience as a hospital administrator – drew up a blue print for Sathya Sai Mission Hospital. There were to be two main blocks in the shape of "O" and "M" along with an out patient and ancillary buildings and service areas.

The drawings and blue prints were taken to Bhagawan by Dr. Punnaivanam and then State President Sri. P.G. Achuthanandam. Swami was very pleased with the idea, created Vibhuthi and sprinkled on the blue prints and gave His blessings to start the project.

I went to a brick manufacturing klin close to Madras and arranged for bricks to be embossed with the name "SAIRAM" on it. The cost for such brick with a bulk order would be less than a rupee. It was decided to print stamps with a picture of this SAIRAM brick. The idea: each devotee visiting a bhajan center would be able to contribute at least one brick for this hospital which would be an edifice of love bearing Bhagawan's name. Booklets were printed with a sheet of ten stamps each. McMillan Press (which had printed Man of Miracles) came forward to waive the upfront payment for the print order and allowed easy installments. In the meanwhile, Sri. Mandradiar, a minister of Govt. of Tamil Nadu had approached Swami for blessing his proposal to build a free hospital in Bhagawan's name at Erode. Bhagawan directed him to join hands with devotees at Coimbatore Hospital Project. Everyone was happy at the progress of events. I got a model of the hospital (6'x6') prepared and took it all the way to Prashanthi Nilayam for blessings. Though Bhagawan did not visit the room (1975) directly, he deputed Dr. Bhagawantham and other elders to have a look at it.

While hectic preparations were going on during Bhagawan's visit to Madras,

January 1976, it was Sri. G. R. Eshwar, another samithi member of Madras, who brought the news that Bhagawan has shelved the plan for Coimbatore hospital with the instruction not to process further. It was shocking news – a bolt from the blue. I could not contain my disappointment. I met Sri. Kasturi who was my mentor and broke down while seeking solace and understanding. I wanted to know why Swami after blessing so profusely and encouraging so much, had decided not to proceed with it. What Sri. Kasturi said that day was a great lesson for me. He said "Doctor, you're disappointed and feel sad because you felt you were doing the project. He knows best as to when where and how to accomplish what He plans. Perhaps He has better plans. Accept His will - that is a mark of true devotion."

When the Super Specialty Hospital was inaugurated in 1991 at Puttaparthi, I could realize the import of Sri. Kasturi's words – In a magnificent way the dream of Sri Sathya Sai Mission Hospital came to fruition. The only hospital of its kind in the entire world and only Bhagawan could accomplish building and commissioning the same in a record time of 6 months.

The compassionate Lord did call and offer me a position in the Super Speciality Hospital. Bhagawan wanted me to train young doctors in Cardiac Anesthesia. I was not fortunate to avail the opportunity because my father had an heart attack and my presence at his bed side was essential at that time.

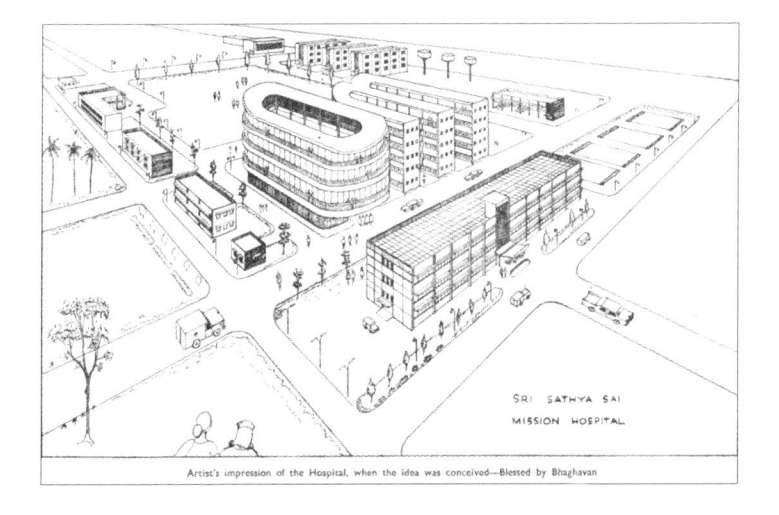

Artist's impression of the Hospital, when the idea was conceived—Blessed by Bhaghavan

Happy Home at Poondamalli

I have crossed by the home for the blind at Poondamalli several times during my childhood and used to wonder how it was inside this red beautiful building. It seemed like a "Red-Fort"(one of the imposing national monuments in New Delhi, and a artifact from Mughal empire circa 1638).

Bhagawan gave me an opportunity to visit this red building. Myself and brother G. Venkatesh – our sevadal leader – reached the place one fine Sunday morning. We had gone there to invite the warden and request him to send a few inmates to participate in the "World Disabled Day" we were celebrating the following Sunday at Sundaram.

We parked in the compound and proceeded towards the building. Strangely, there were no notice boards to indicate the entrance or where the office was. We entered the building through one of the doors and found ourselves in a large courtyard with wooden steps leading to the first floor. The place was buzzing with activity. There was a line of little girls taking their turn to receive coconut oil in the cup of their palms, giggling and laughing and bubbling with happiness since it was their head bath day. We also found a couple of boys holding hands and coming down the steps – two at a time – discussing about the breakfast they just had. There was another group of four to five boys holding on to a transistor and commenting on Gavaskar's century and all the fringes of the exciting game of cricket.

All of them were totally oblivious to our presence because they are visually challenged inmates.

As I was discussing with Venkatesh whether we should enquire from one of the cricket fans, the youngest of them recognized my voice and came towards me enquiring "what doctor, when did you come. Can I help you!!"

Apparently I had seen him at Saikrupa and treated him for his fever and cough the previous Sunday. How God compensates by giving sharpness in one faculty while the other is ineffective is a marvel and a testament to His limitless compassion.

When we expressed our desire to meet their warden, he at once offered his hand and asked us to follow him.

Holding my hands, he quickly took us to the warden's room through a maze of corridors and steps all without board or signs, and introduced us to the warden and even fetched two tumblers of water for us. We were awestruck and amazed that our two pair of eyes(mine fortified with glasses) was of no use in that building.

The mirth, happiness and joy found inside those walls were so profound that there is nothing in the outside world that could match it. We realized the significance of calling these children "differently abled" and thanked Bhagawan for this eye opener.

> "I know the agitations of your heart and its aspirations, but you don't know my heart. I react to the pain your undergo and joy you feel, for I am in your heart. I am the dweller in the temple of every heart. Do not loose contact and company, for it is only when the lump of coal is in contact with live ember that it can also become a live ember. Cultivate nearness with me in the heart and you will be rewarded. Then you too will acquire a fraction of the supreme love. This is a great chance. Be confident that all will be liberated. Many hesitate to believe that things will improve: that life will be happy for all and full of joy, and the golden age will recur. Let me assure you that this Dharma swarupa, this divine body, has not come in vain. It will succeed in warding off the crises that has come upon humanity." – Baba

Section 2 –

Expanding Medical Service

Bhagawan's Visit to SaiKrupa

3rd September 1980 was a red lettered day for SaiKrupa. Bhagawan visited SaiKrupa and spent nearly an hour of His time. He went through all sections, saw the display boards, blessed the badges for doctors and volunteers and distributed prasadam to everyone before accepting Aarthi.

We had kept a framed picture of Bhagawan with a stethoscope at the altar. We wanted a picture of Swami looking through the microscope. We had planted two photographers, one in the lab and another from behind the partition perched on a table to take a picture of Swami. As Bhagawan was going around, I requested Him to look through the microscope so that we will be blessed with a picture. Bhagawan laughed and touched my chest and adviced me to look into the microscope there(heart) and find Him. All arrangements to capture a picture of Bhagwan looking through microscope failed – happily and not miserably. For I had been blessed with the divine touch and a profound lesson in the use of heart to capture Him permanently.

Lord never forgets the wishes of his devotees. Years later when I received a complimentary copy of a book written by Dr. Bhat (Considered as Father of Urology in South India), I found a picture in it where Swami is looking through the flourescent microscope!!

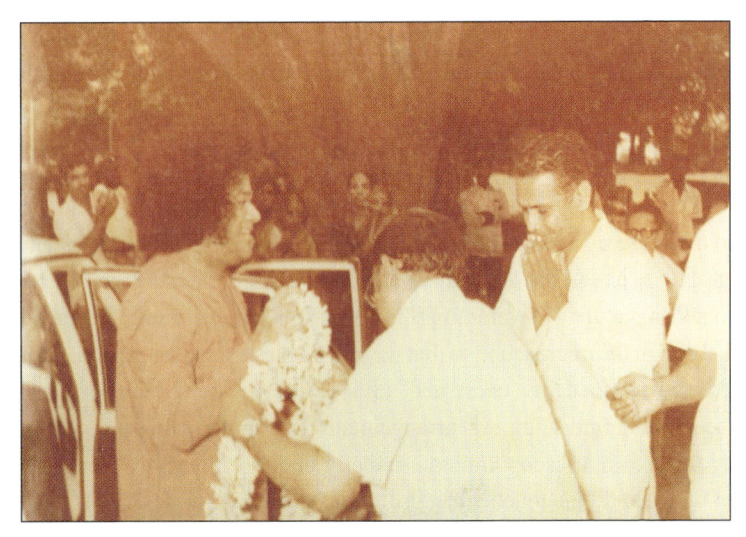

Bhagawan arrives on His first visit to SaiKrupa – Sep. 3, 1980

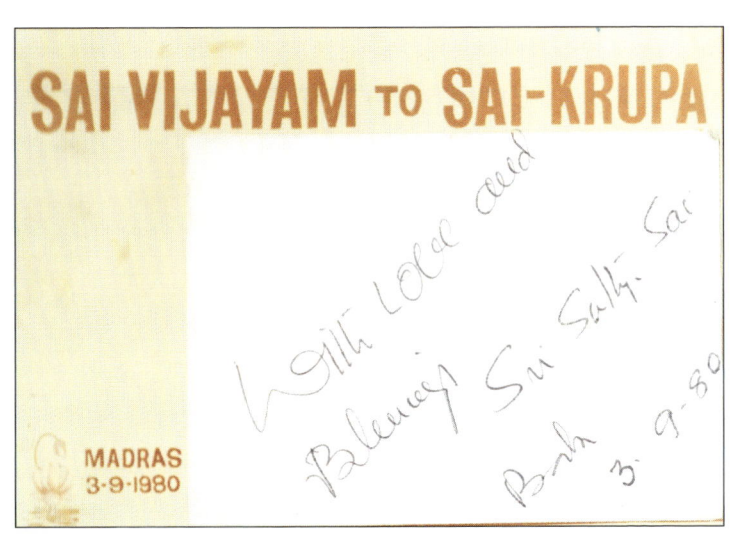

Bhagawan graciously autographed the album of His first visit to Sai Krupa.
We continue to bask in that eternal love that He alone is capable of showering.

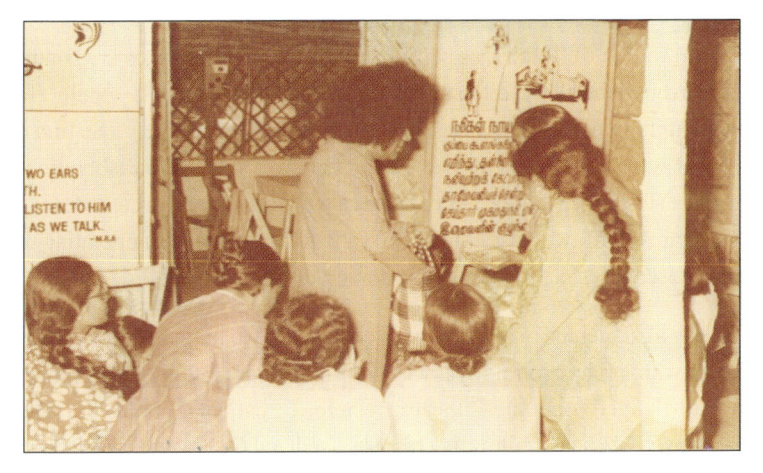

Bhagawan graciously distributes vibuthi packets to
doctors at SaiKrupa – Sep. 3, 1980

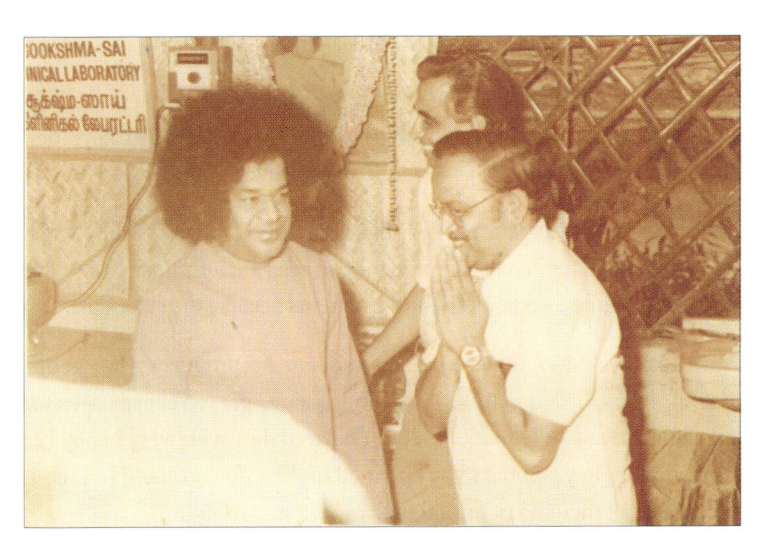

Though I failed to get Bhagawan to see through the microscope,
He touched my heart and said "See me here". It's a profound lesson not
only for me but for all of humanity - to seek Him in our hearts.

To my right is Dr. C.S. Lakshminarayana – Prof. and Head of Dept. of
Microbiology, Madras Medical College.

Abbotsbury Transforms into Eye Hospital

In the Tamil month of "Aadi", as per local tradition, no marriages are conducted. Therefore Abbottsbury wasn't booked for wedding during this month. Taking advantage of its availability, major service activities were planned. The first major activity that was carried was an eye camp. This was done in collaboration with Aravind Eye Hospital, Madurai. Aravind has a well organized eye camp team. They move in a caravan of two buses and three vans fully loaded with operating tables, lamps, microscopes, sterile instruments, drapes, dressings, etc.

Abbottsbury also seemed to be ideally suited venue. Two main halls served as male and female wards. The central foyer was partitioned, air conditioned and sterilized into a full-fledged operation theatre where 6 patients could be operated simultaneously. Mats and pillows were purchased and 6'x3' were ear marked with aisle space for moving trolleys and gaps inter connecting rows. Wing Commander Dr. Ramanath was a volunteer at SaiKrupa - he was able to mobilize his friends from the Indian Air Force(IAF) to dig and prepare make-shift sanitary facilities as a supplement to cover large number of patients along with the attendees and the volunteer force.

Meticulous details were worked out and the functioning of the camp went on very smoothly for the entire one week period by Sai Grace. The food arrangements for all and morning and evening bhajans were also organized.

On Day 1 the crowd was jam packed, nearly a 1000. Nearly 180 patients were selected and operated upon on Day 2 and looked after for a further 6 days. The love with which the volunteers attended to these patients became the talk of the town.

To my surprise, I found a famous music director and his producer who got operated at the camp. They had quietly entered the queue, got screened, selected and operated upon like any other patient. They declared they were very happy lying on the mat provided. They wanted to be operated in the safety of Sai Eye Camp. That was the hallmark of their devotion and faith in Swami.

This was the starting point and its echo was felt throughout Tamil Nadu. All the district level Samithis also wanted to conduct such eye camps and a very good rapport was created with Aravind Eye Hospital who were very willing to come and serve anywhere the Sai Organisation conducted an eye camp. Bhagawan was pleased immensely with this service and provided Tamil Nadu with a chance to conduct an Eye Camp at Prashanthi Nilayam.

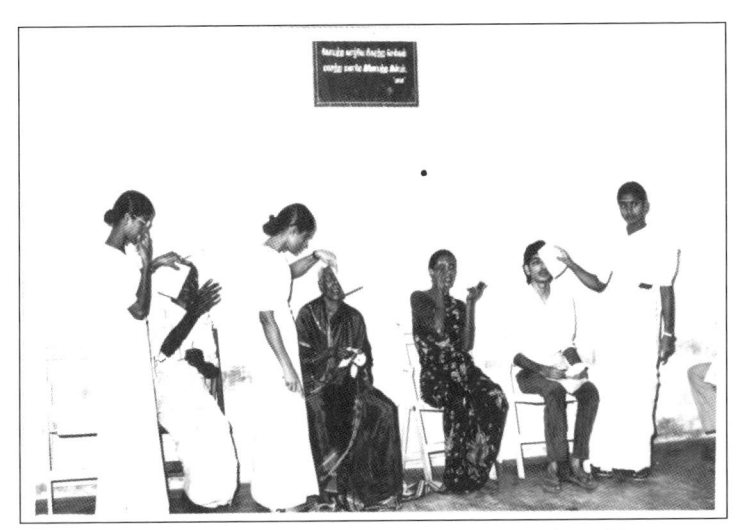

Vision exam for patients at eye camp – conducted by technicians from Arvind Eye Hospital

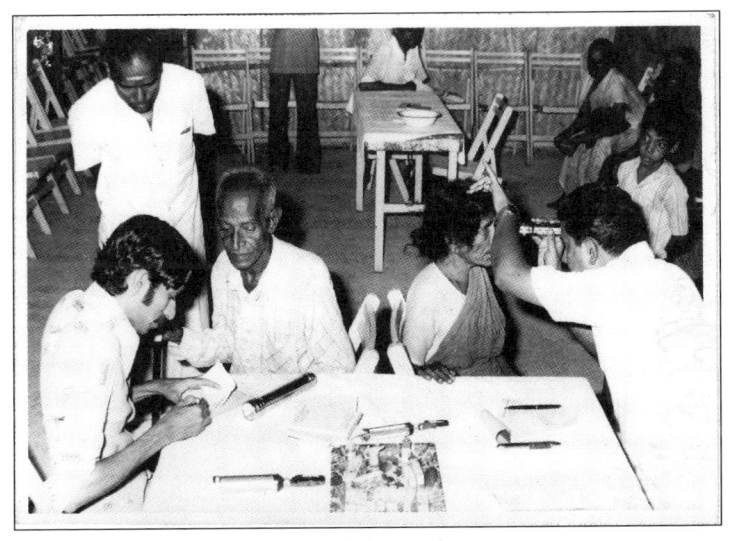

Opthomologists examining patients at eye camp

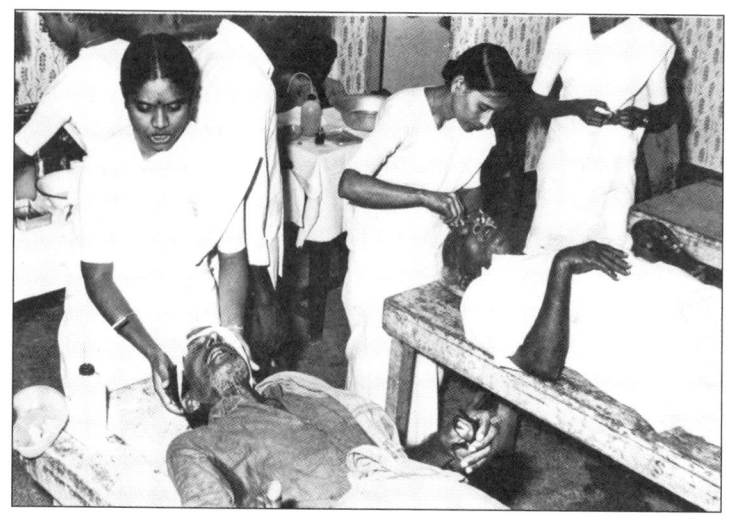

Post Operative care for patients at eye camp

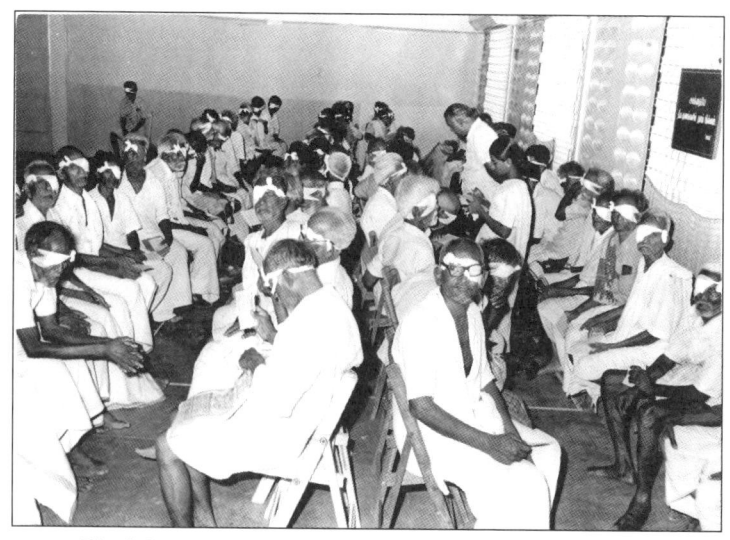

Final day – patients waiting for bandages to be removed

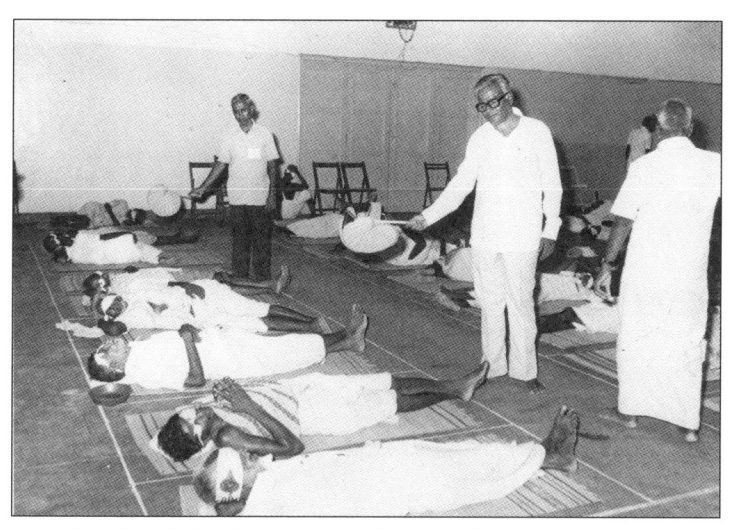

Sai Care: Volunteers (Seva Dal) ensured that every patient was cared for in a loving manner

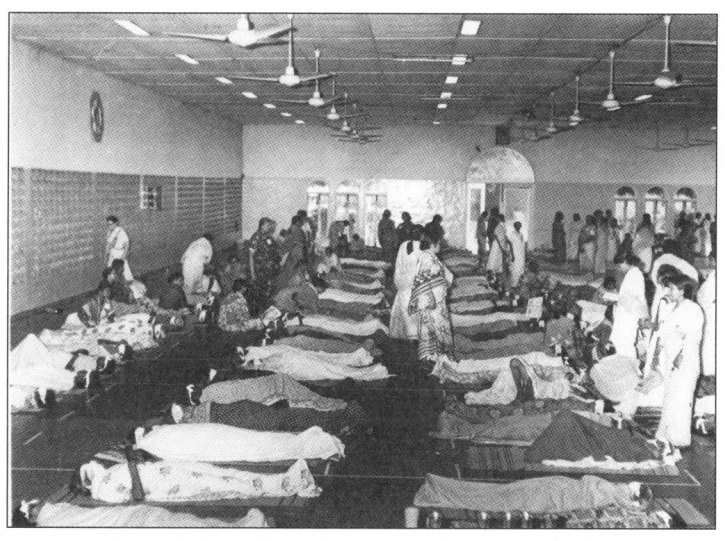

Large hall at Abbotsbury converted to a ward for eye camp patients by Sevadals

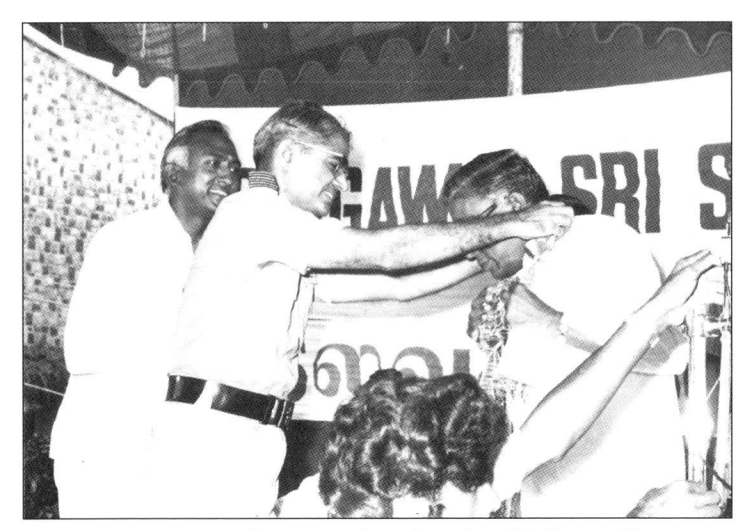

Wing Commander Ramnath welcoming chief guest Hon. Minister Thiru R.M. Veerappan of Tamil Nadu Govt.

Spare 2 Tablets for My Grace

Sathya Sai Trust had acquired 4 tenements built by Slum Clearance board for rent (Subsequently purchased) at Anna Nagar for the Sai Samithi. Dr. Susheela Sambamoorthy along with a team of volunteers started a medical service at the premises. Thus 'Anna Nagar SaiKrupa' came in to existence. The name stuck on not only in other free clinics in Tamil Nadu but many centers across the globe wherever our volunteers have gone and served have been named as SaiKrupa.

Bhagawan visited Anna Nagar SaiKrupa in the early 80's and spent nearly an hour going around. He was amused by the fabricated Dental chair and commented that it is nicely done but the gargling tray and spitting bin was on the wrong side. He also blessed the camphor tableting unit installed there. During the weekdays, manufacturing Sundaram Brand Camphor tablets was one of the activities at the centre. He blessed the doctors and signed the OP register and the specially designed health check up cards. Sri. Menon requested Bhagawan to advice the doctors. Swami readily agreed and talked to the doctors for about 10 minutes. He advised them to concentrate on preventive aspects and teach patients about proper hygiene and nutrition. He was critical of the heavy usage of antibiotics. He said chloromycin, terramycin– are all sins.

Allowing the body to heal itself without dumping antibiotics for every small ailment is the right thing to do – according to Bhagawan. And as a parting salvo, He said "Where you have to give 10 tablets give 8. Spare two so that my grace can also act!!" He concedes 80% credit to doctors and retains 20% for His grace in the cure of a patient. He mentioned it in such a humble and soft tone – a subtle reminder to the egoistic doctors that God's grace is also necessary for affecting a cure.

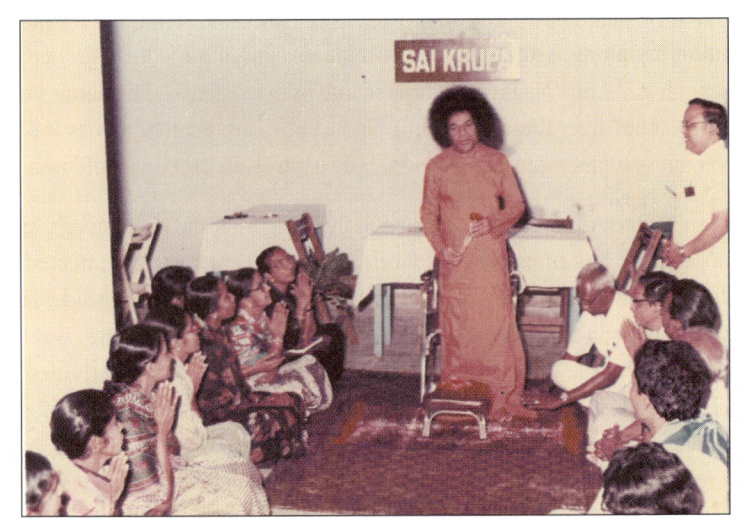

Bhagawan with doctors at SaiKrupa

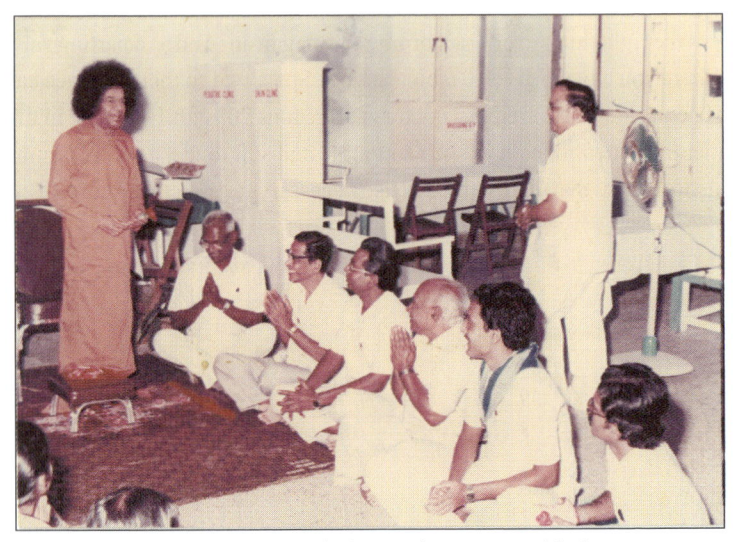

Bhagawan shares a light hearted moment with doctors

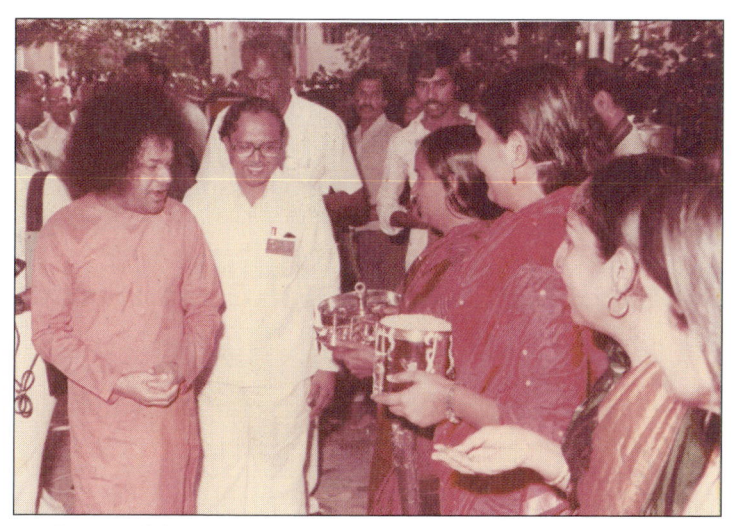

Ceremonial welcome to Bhagawan at Anna Nagar Sai Samithi

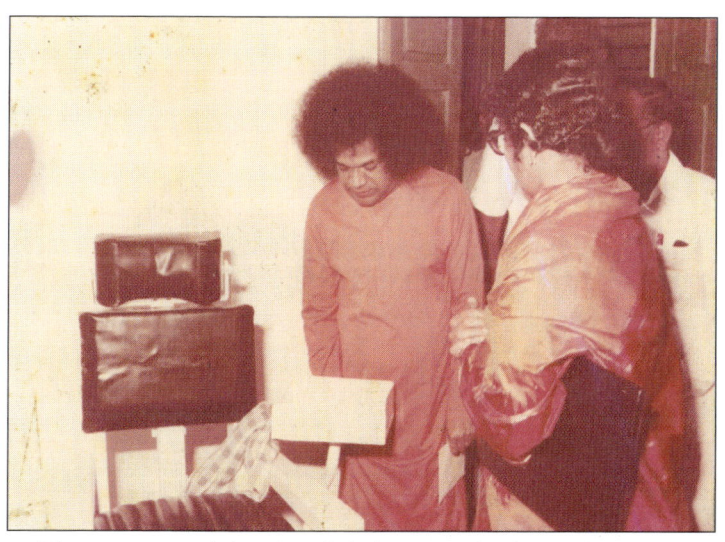

Bhagawan examining dental chair. Dr. Susheela Sambamurthy, convenor of Anna Nagar SaiKrupa is seen explaining to Bhagawan

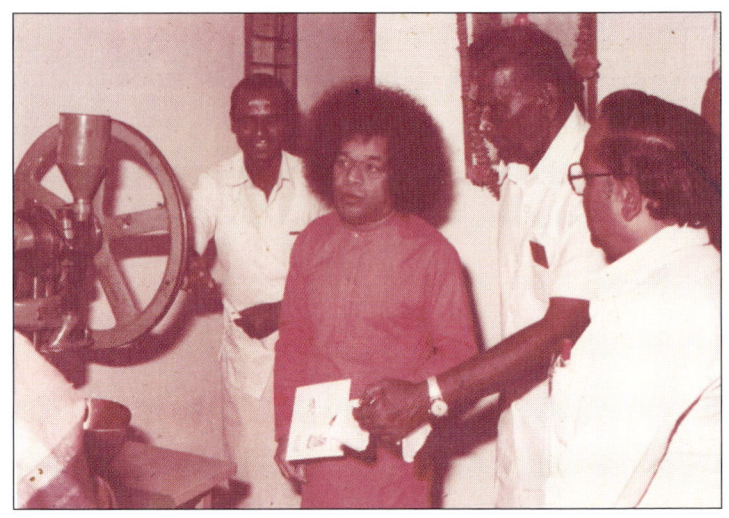

Bhagawan tours Camphor manufacturing facility in Anna Nagar Sai Samithi

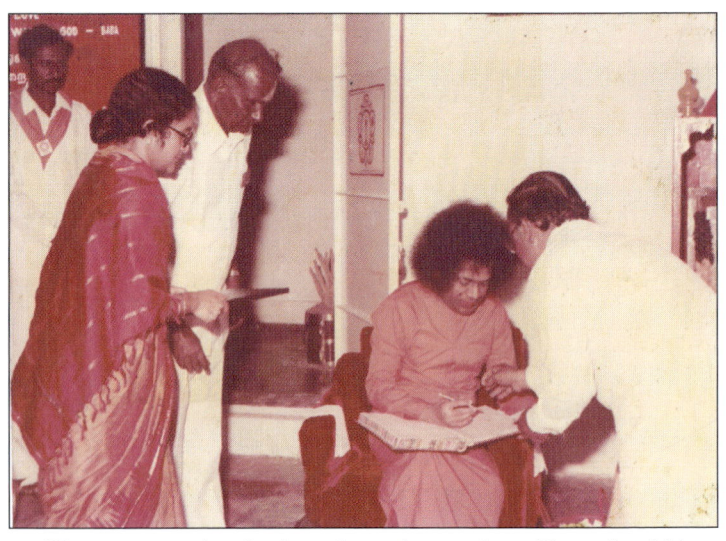

Bhagawan graciously signs the register at Anna Nagar Samithi

Bringing Care to Senior Citizens

"Nobody listens to us" – this is a common complaint from senior citizens. Aches and pains are common. Busy offsprings do not find time or postpone getting medical attention and care for them. We decided for once, we will make fuss, attend to every physical complaint and provide relief.

For the first time in the city a major camp for the elderly was conducted at Abbottsbury. Nearly 120 doctors and specialists offered their service in this 6 hour Sunday Camp. About 200 Sai Volunteers (men and women) offered their labour of love and with Bhgawan's grace established SaiKrupa at Abbottsbury as a landmark for medical seva.

The Health minister who visited the camp was amazed to find that facilities were created for all the specialists at the same place so nicely. He said such a thing did not exist even in a major teaching hospital in the city. Walking sticks, cervical collars, eye glasses, etc. were provided free of cost on prescription from doctors. Dental department attended to all dental problems and with arrangement with Raga's Dental College, free dentures were also provided to the needy. The orthopedic department was the busiest. There was routine cancer screenings performed by about half a dozen gynecologists. Diabetologists with the lab support screened all patients.

All elderly patients were received with a smile, made to sit comfortably, and served a cup of hot tea as they were registered. Along with the OP ticket, an empty container was also given to collect urine sample for albumin and sugar test at the lab before entering the main hall for consultation. Thus the main problem of crowd management, especially the elderly, was solved viz. (1) empty stomach and (2) full bladder. All had their BP checked by the physicians and if found necessary they could consult a cardiologist who had an ECG machine with him. All were seen by the eye specialist and dental surgeon. Other specialists like ENT, General Surgeon, Neurologist, Skin and Geriatric specialists were available to see referred cases. The X – Ray van was stationed at the portico with facilities for developing the films and reporting by radiologists. It was like a mini hospital, especially for the elderly. Nearly 600 elderly people availed the facilities of the Sai Geriatric camp. In reporting this event, local press was all praise for the arrangements and loving service.

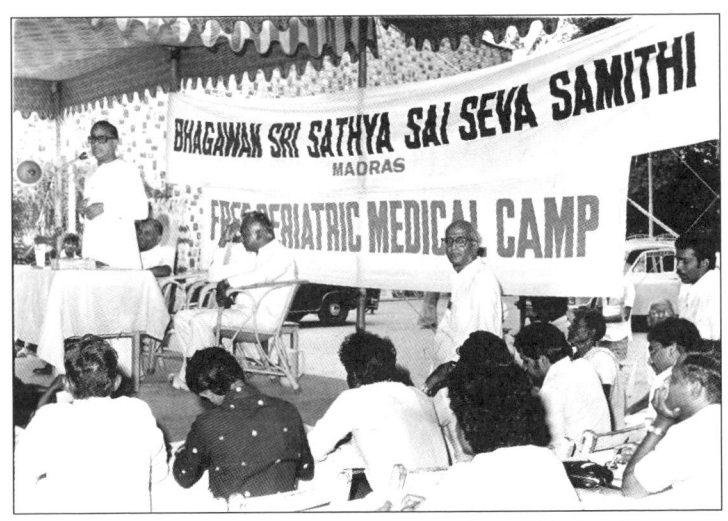

Dr. Hande – minister for health, govt. of Tamil Nadu, gives a keynote address at inauguration of Geriatric Camp

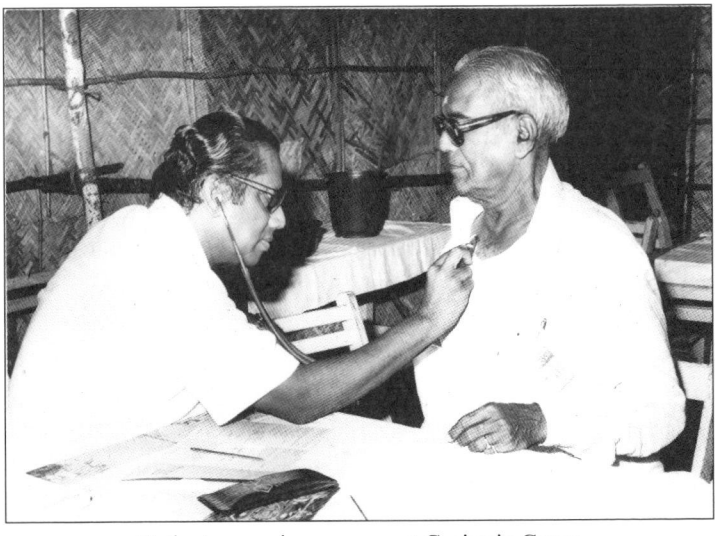

Patient exam in progress at Geriatric Camp

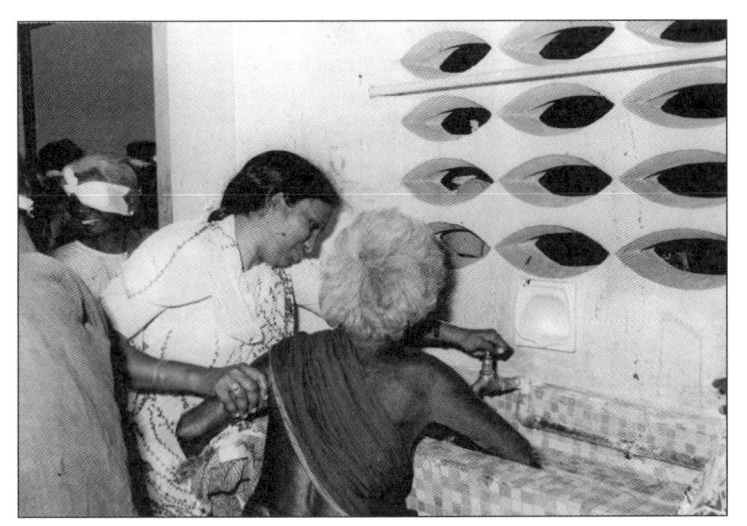

Love and care provided by Mahila volunteers at Eye camp

All India Seva Training – Prashanthi Nilayam

Bhagawan graciously agreed to allow devotees to celebrate his 60th birthday spread over 3 years. 1983 November was celebrated as Balavikas Year and programs were conducted by Balavikas children. 1984 November was to be celebrated as Sevadal Year, highlighting seva activities. Each state highlighted the activity in which it had specialized and was directed to train All India Sevadal Volunteers in that particular activity. There were nearly a dozen identified activities.

Tamil Nadu was assigned the task of training volunteers in conducting Eye Camps. SaiKrupa which was assigned this duty had prepared an 'Eye Camp Training Manual' and copies of the same were distributed to volunteers from all over India. Dr. C. Rajkumar, Dr. Shiva Subramaniam and myself conducted the training classes. I was also given the task of organizing the Tamil Nadu stall in the international exhibition on seva activities. Tamil Nadu stall was decorated as a temple with a gopuram cut out on the top. Photographs of all activities, including medical seva, were displayed. Bhagawan blessed this stall with His visit and evinced keen interest by viewing all material in great detail.

> "It is significant to note that those who live on vegetarian food are less prone to diseases whereas non-vegetarians are more subject to diseases. The reason is animal food is incompatible with the needs of human body"– Baba

Bhagawan's Advice on Eye Camps

Once Bhagwan asked the doctors assembled what is the success rate at eye camp. We proudly announced that it was 98 – 99%. Bhagawan's comment was that it may be a great achievement for you to claim 99% success rate but that one patient would say "I was operated at Sai Baba eye camp and I lost my vision."

Bhagawan's advice was to henceforth only screen the patients at the camp site, but have surgery done in a regular hospital.

This was a eye opener – it revealed to us the perfection that He embodies. He doesn't want anyone left behind. His immense love and concern for that one patient inspired us and showed how medical care is to be delivered.

In accordance with Bhagawan's command, screening is done and cases are referred to hospitals for follow up care.

> "Meat is alright for those who concentrate on the body and want to have strength. But for spiritual aspirants it is not good. Dirty thoughts come with fish. Although fish is always in water, it has a bad smell."– Baba

They Wanted to do All the Walking

The surgical polio camp was one of the most heart warming camps conducted by the Sai Organisation at Abbottsbury. Dr. Vyagreswarudu, an eminent Ortho Surgeon who had taken up surgical treatment for polio affected children as a mission in his life was invited along with his team - Dr. Bapi Raju, Dr. Murthy and 6 others - to come to SaiKrupa. They brought with them all the required surgical equipment. The AC operation theatre with full infrastructure, along with anesthesia services and autoclaving facilities were provided by the Sai Organization. Both halls at Abbotsbury were converted into wards as done during the eye camp.

It was sheer Sai Grace that I.C.I. factory which had kept on hold manufacturing of "Halothane" a wonder anesthesia drug which makes the crying children smoothly go to sleep without the poke of an injection – resumed its production and the very first two bottles (Rs. 5,000 each) were given as donation for the camp. The surgical team was experiencing the ease with which surgery could be performed for the first time in this camp. Facilities were available for 6 surgeries at a time with anesthesia machines, gas and oxygen cylinders and halothane vaporizers. 4 qualified anesthesiologists provided their services.

The publicity for the camp was taken up by the railway unions(comprised of Sai devotees) and posters were pasted in all stations of Southern Railway. It was a tough job of controlling the crowd of about 800 children with their attendants at Abbottsbury on Day 1. 96 selected cases were operated upon on Day 2. They were discharged on Day 7 after removal of stitches and measurements taken for fitting calipers and shoes. All operated cases were asked to report after a month. On that day the team returned with the calipers and fitted them on the operated leg. The children were taught to walk between rows of benches and chairs. It was a heart warming sight to see the excitement in the children. They would not leave the place. They wanted to do all the walking they had missed in their earlier years. For the parents, sight of their children in an erect position taking their steps without being obliged to crawl at the ground level was a very satisfying experience. Thus Sai Love made it possible to overcome a crippling disease with surgery and rehabilitation. Dignity of the child and the family was restored in the process.

The Health Minister who inaugurated the camp was so impressed that he deputed the Director of Medical Education and the Director of Medical Services to see the camp. Polio is a neglected condition and nowhere facilities are available to attend to them in a scale at which Sai Organization had created and offered the service totally free of cost and with so much Love. The Press hailed it as a major service project.

Because of the large number of children requiring this service, similar camps were planned and conducted at Neyveli and Coimbatore by the Sai Organization. In total, 400 children who used to crawl on all their fours, were able to walk in erect posture due to surgery and the support of calipers. It restored dignity and provided a near normal quality of life to these children.

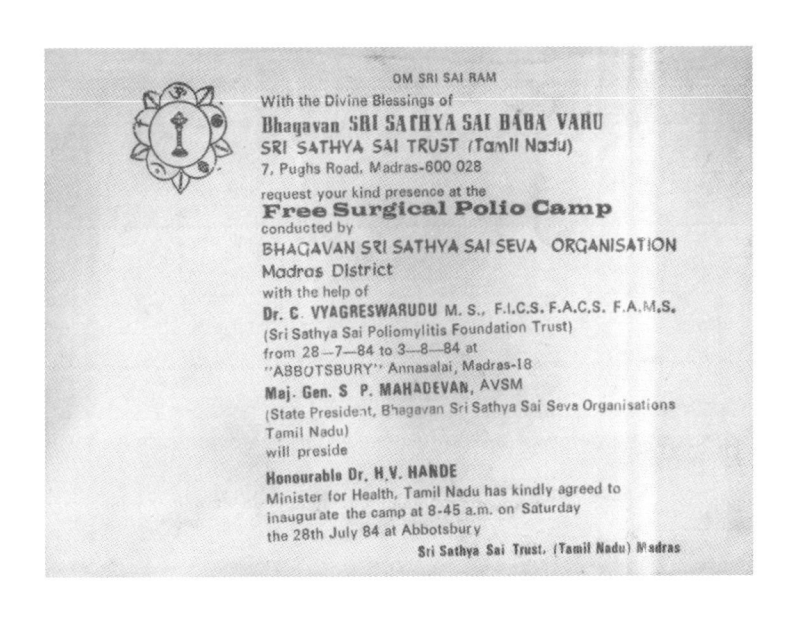

> OM SRI SAI RAM
>
> With the Divine Blessings of
>
> **Bhagavan SRI SATHYA SAI BABA VARU**
> SRI SATHYA SAI TRUST (Tamil Nadu)
> 7, Pughs Road, Madras-600 028
>
> request your kind presence at the
> **Free Surgical Polio Camp**
> conducted by
> BHAGAVAN SRI SATHYA SAI SEVA ORGANISATION
> Madras District
> with the help of
> **Dr. C. VYAGRESWARUDU** M. S., F.I.C.S. F.A.C.S. F.A.M.S.
> (Sri Sathya Sai Poliomylitis Foundation Trust)
> from 28—7—84 to 3—8—84 at
> "ABBOTSBURY" Annasalai, Madras-18
>
> **Maj. Gen. S P. MAHADEVAN**, AVSM
> (State President, Bhagavan Sri Sathya Sai Seva Organisations Tamil Nadu)
> will preside
>
> **Honourable Dr. H.V. HANDE**
> Minister for Health, Tamil Nadu has kindly agreed to inaugurate the camp at 8-45 a.m. on Saturday the 28th July 84 at Abbotsbury
>
> Sri Sathya Sai Trust, (Tamil Nadu) Madras

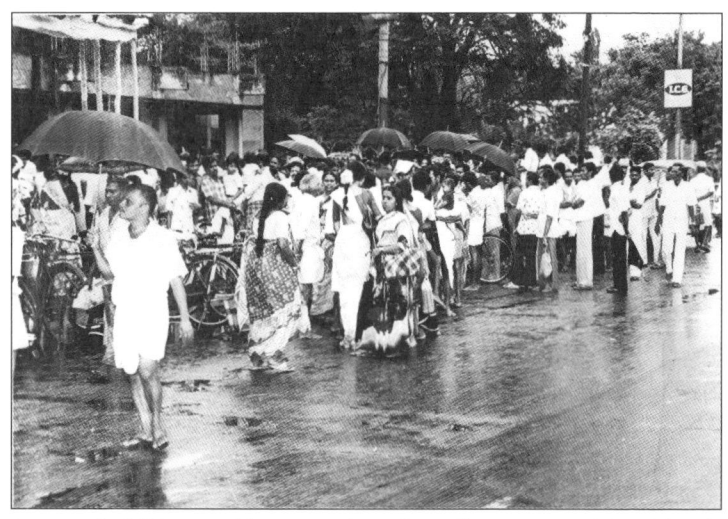

Patients and children waiting to register for polio camp outside Abbotsbury

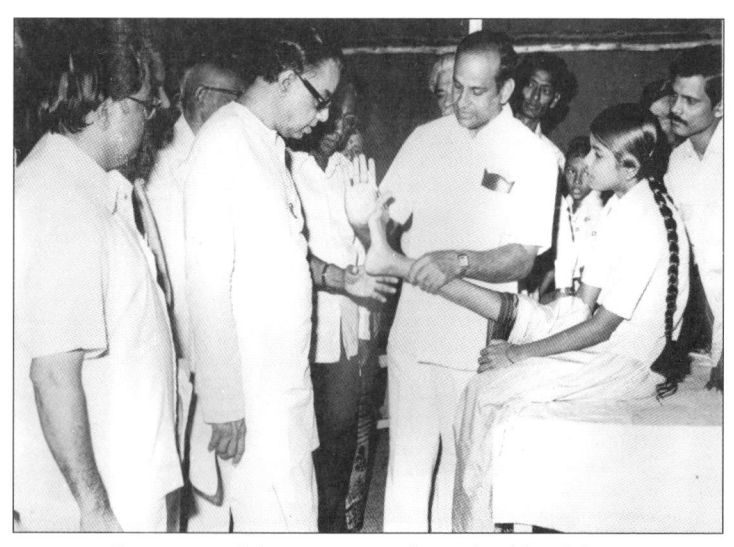

Surgeon explains treatment plan to health minister
Dr. Hande of Tamil Nadu Govt.

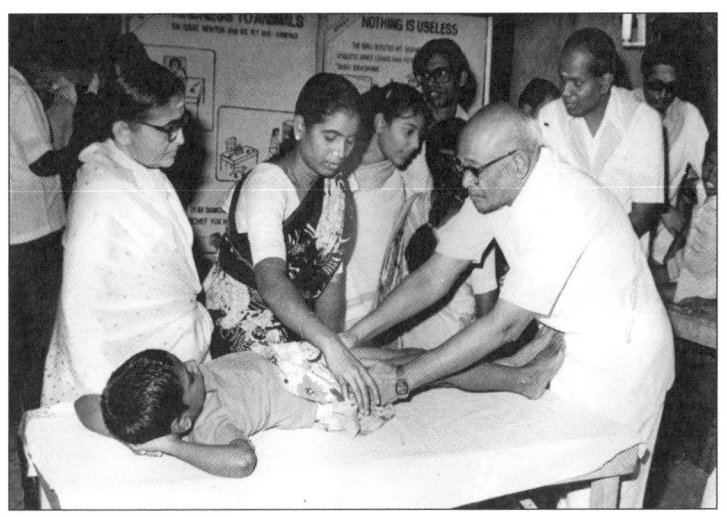

Orthopedic surgeon Dr. Vyagreswaradu examines a patient screened for surgery

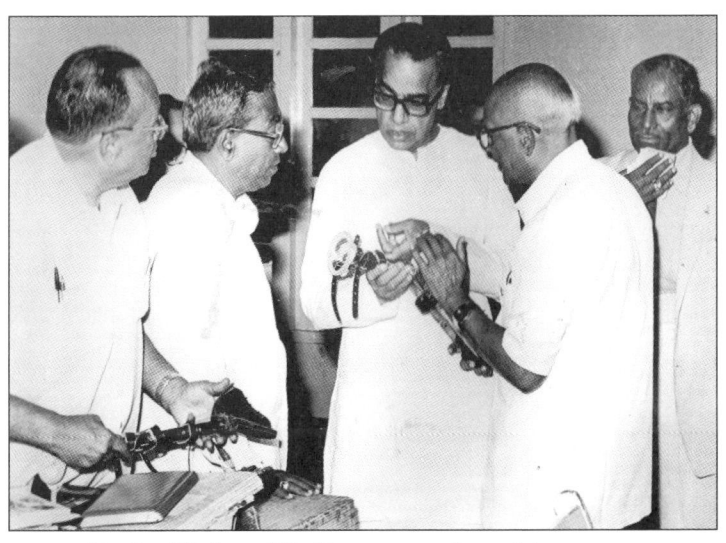

Dr. Bapi Raju and Dr. Vyagreswaradu explain process
of fitting calipers, post surgery, to Dr. Hande

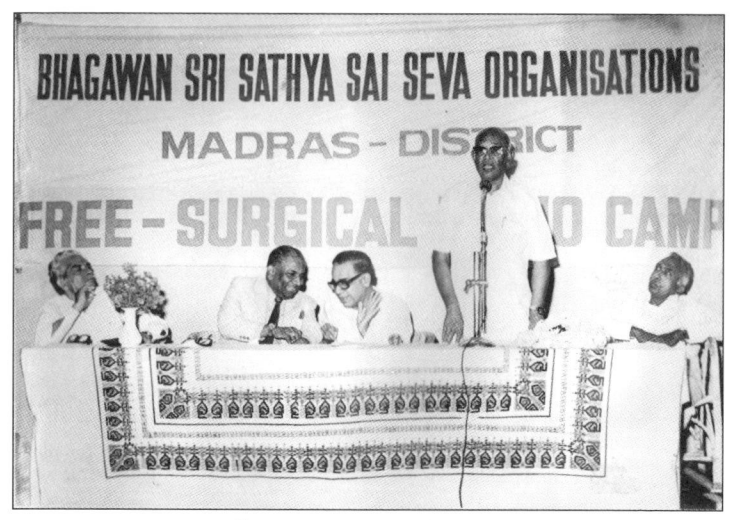

Polio Camp Inaugural Function

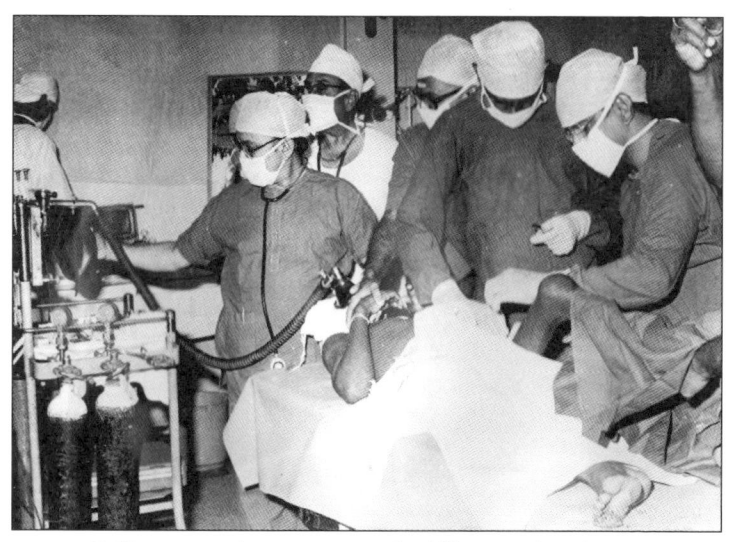

Polio surgery in progress, makeshift operating theater created by doctors and volunteers at Abbotsbury

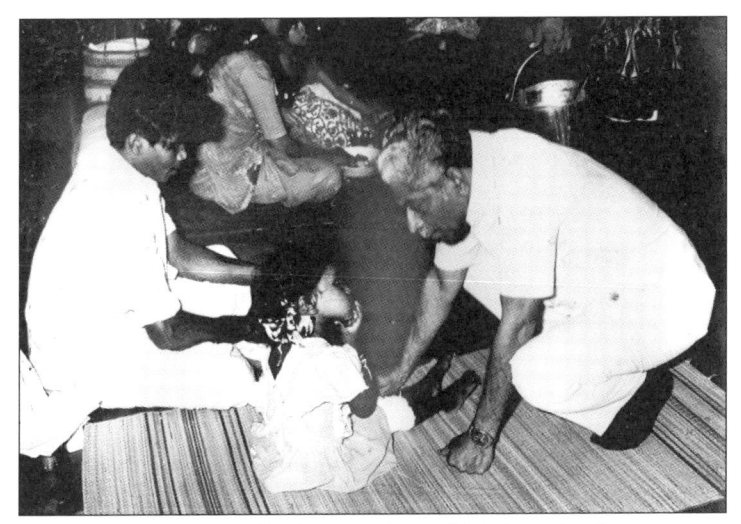

Then Madras district president of Sai Organization,
Sri. M. Basker, makes loving enquires of patient recovering from polio surgery

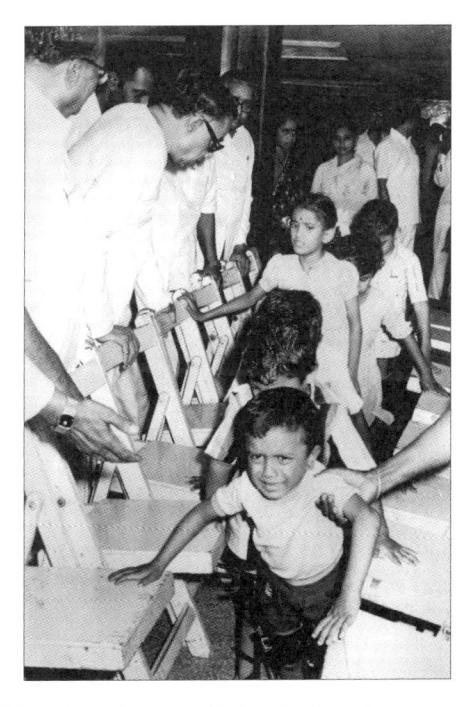

Children learning to walk for the first time post surgery.
For children and parents, it was a miracle come true

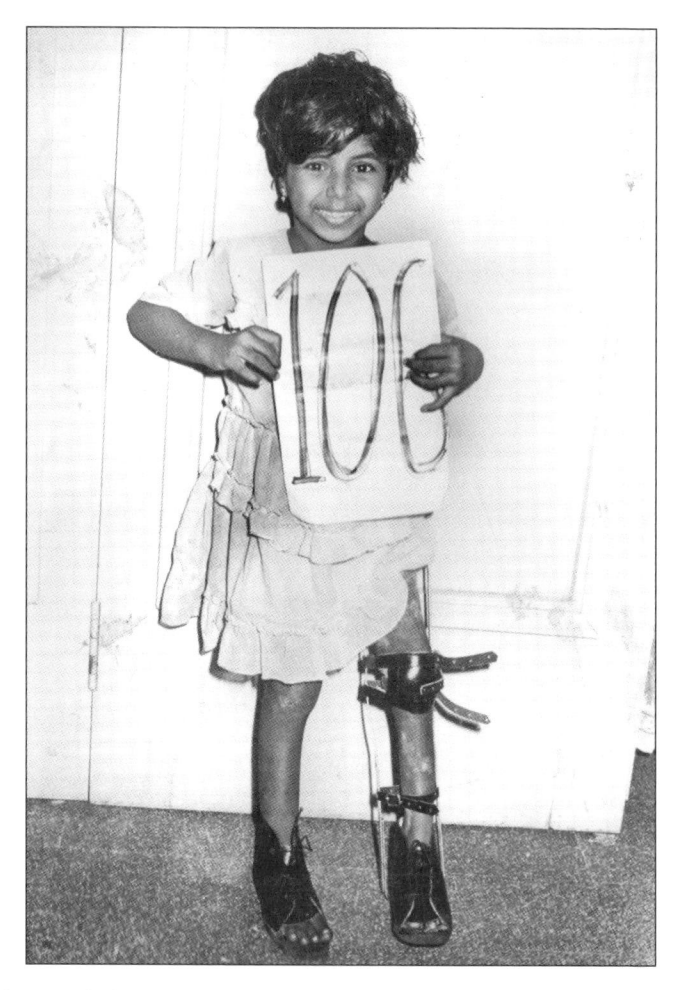

Happiness at being able to walk and move about is visible in this child's face

The Lord came down as man to show us how to walk on the royal path that leads to His abode. His joy knows no bounds when He sees us walking on this path.

Dental Camp

A major dental camp was also organized by SaiKrupa in the ground floor of the huge 8 storey building coming up in its compound, in collaboration with the Rural Dentistry wing of the Madras Dental College. In total, 12 dental chairs (half of them brand new units and the rest of them borrowed from local practitioners) were installed. One full automated dental couch with ancillary equipment, with X – ray facility were also installed by a company free of charge. Nearly 600 patients were attended to with extractions, filling, scaling, cleaning, etc. and patients booked at the college for making dentures available to them – the cost of dentures was borne by the Sai Organization. This was one of the camps which produced very satisfying outcomes. About 200 volunteers participated in this one day camp at Abbottsbury.

Though regular dental chairs were installed with temporary power connection, water connection could not be given. Make shift arrangements were made with blue color plastic buckets with clean water and plastic tumbler. The patients were asked to pick up water to rinse and gargle and allowed to spit into a red colored water bucket held by volunteers. It was a sight to see: lady volunteers clad in silk sarees who typically had domestic help to attend on chores at home, happily doing this service of collecting the waste water soiled with blood and washings.

Extraction of painful teeth, filing of cavities, cleaning and scaling, thereby removing foul odour from the mouth provided dramatic and immediate relief. Many patients were happy that they could once again chew and eat normal food.

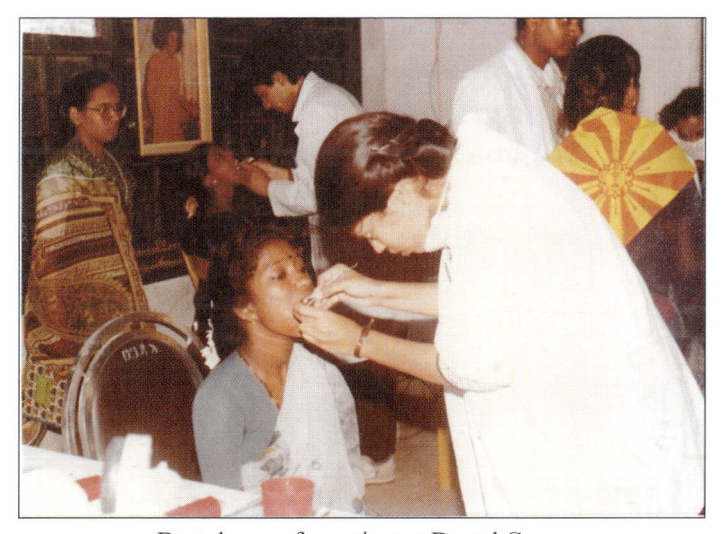

Dental exam for patient at Dental Camp

WHO Team Visits SaiKrupa

A W.H.O. team was tasked with visiting Asian countries to study infrastructure available in developing countries for providing medicare. Africa was insisting on proper buildings and equipment for rural dispensaries. There was a big gap between funds available and the requirements put forth by African authorities. The team had heard about SaiKrupa which functioned in a thatched structure with minimal facilities catering to a large number of patients and with very good outcomes. They were wonderstruck to learn that the entire workforce of doctors, paramedics and general workers were offering service free of cost and discharging their duties with so much of love.

One African gentleman of the team was found to be going around both inside and outside of thatched structure several times and then going and sitting on a chair and weeping profusely. When asked by the doctors about the cause of his emotional breakdown he revealed that he had dreamt seeing this very same thatched structure with a bamboo grill exactly as found in SaiKrupa. He described how a man in orange robe and an African hairdo was talking so kindly to all people sitting on the benches and blessing each by placing his hands on their heads. He had seen this dream vividly atleast 8 or 10 times during the previous weeks while in Africa and was wondering why and where this place was. When he saw Swami's picture on the altar at SaiKrupa he was able to instantly recognize him.

All who heard him were dumbfounded and overwhelmed by Bhagawan's love. Bhagawan's ways are inscrutable… His immediate purpose seems to be to provide direction and guidance for the African gentleman; indirectly and through the very same set of dreams, He revealed His visits and blessings for SaiKrupa. Bhagawan likens His ways to that of striking one ball in billiards – whilst it appears that only one ball has been struck, it moves many other balls on the table towards the goal.

Silver Jubilee of Sai Organization

Bhagawan always puts emphasis on prevention of ailments. In view of this, a major health education exhibition was organized. The display of boards was organized under shamianas in the Sundaram compound, which was inaugurated by the chief secretary of Govt. of Tamil Nadu. The meeting portion was held under a pandal in the play ground in the SaiKrupa complex. There were arrangements for nutrition demonstration by Mahilas. They taught the value of balanced diet and how tasty dishes could be prepared from Ragi(millet) etc.

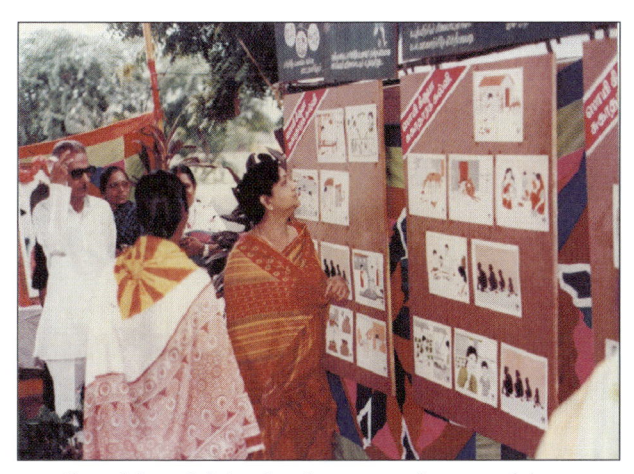

Sevadal explaining hygiene procedures to visitors

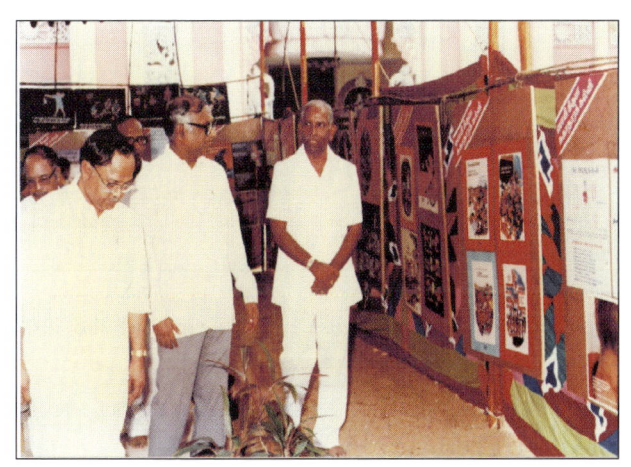

Chief Secretary to Govt. of Tamil Nadu evincing keen interest on preventive aspects of health

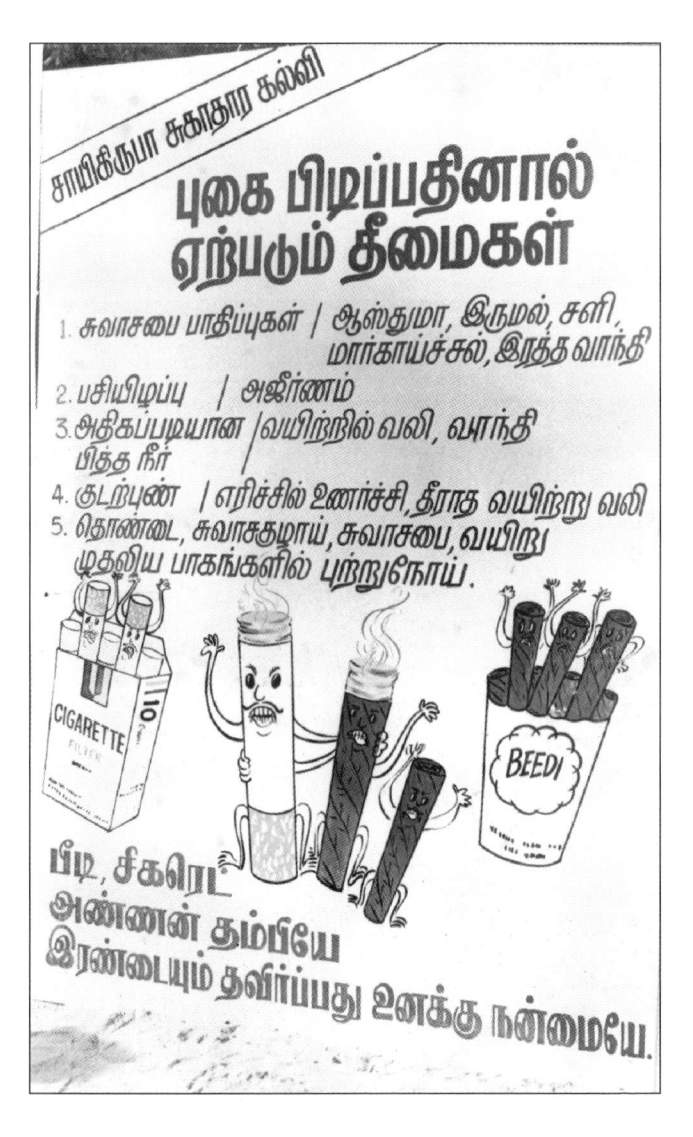

Raising awareness on health issues caused by smoking and drinking

SaiKrupa on the Move

During 1984 Abbottsbury was sold and we had to vacate. Though Bhagawan always cautions not to get attached to worldy things which are transient – My attachment to Abbottsbury was very deep with so many memories and thrills of Sai Seva and the ever lasting joy of Sai Darshan and His presence and discourses during several occasions – it was with sadness we bid farewell to Abbottsbury, and relocated SaiKrupa at Rameshwaram Road in T. Nagar, Chennai. It was also a fairly big complex with multiple small flats and a parking lot. It originally belonged to Dr. Dhairyam which had been transferred to the Trust. Different departments started functioning in different rooms on the ground and first floor. Patients' waiting area was managed with a shamiana. Over a period of 3 to 4 weeks more patients started reporting and there was an average attendance of 250 patients every Sunday.

Health Education and Pediatric Screening

A Pediatric Camp was organized in the new location. Details of proper nutrition and immunization program with charts/slides, boards were provided. Dr. Giridharagopal, Dr. Kumari Menon, Dr. Rama Devi, and other Specialists attended this camp. Health Education Boards were also displayed. After this camp, more and more patients in the new area started utilizing SaiKrupa services.

Close to Sundaram

Since Rameswaram Road property was also being sold, SaiKrupa was relocated to a building about 450 Sq.feet in size, built by the Trust in the compound of Chennapuri Annadhana Samajam, Pughs Road – very close to Sundaram . Sundaram is one of three spiritual centers established by Bhagawan. First of these spiritual centers was Sathyam in Mumbai, followed by Sivam in Hyderabad; Sai Krupa almost became an annexe to Sundaram.

This relocation was in the early part of 1986. It was a small hall with one room for the Lab. Temporary partition and screens were used to bifurcate work areas. Though space was a big constraint inside, the huge compound could buffer our needs. We were permitted to use foyer of the school building and the warden's room for additional space. We had to shift furniture and equipment back in to our building at close of work and lock it up till the following Sunday. Sri. Srinivasan has been in-charge of this duty from day 1.

SaiKrupa began to serve patients from nearby slums: Sai Nagar – the first slum adopted by the Sai organization. SaiKrupa also started to attend on medical needs on a regular basis, for about 250 children staying in the hostel of Chennapuri Anandana Samajam – in the same compound. Regular Narayan seva is organized for the visiting patients every Sunday. By Bhagawan's grace SaiKrupa has continued to this day at this very location.

Annadana Samajam for Eye Camp

Since the school at Annadana Samajam was closed for summer vacation, space was available. Taking advantage of space availability, an Eye Camp was organized. The same team from Arvind Eye Hospital arrived with their staff and equipment. They screened 800 and operated on 96 cataract patients. Prescription eye glasses were provided to students and other children who needed corrective lens. Gradually, activity of organizing Eye camps spread all over Tamil Nadu. For Bhagawan's 70th Birth Day (1995) Tamil Nadu dedicated 7,000 cataract operations at the divine lotus feet (70,000 patients were screened).

As per directions of Bhagawan, during subsequent eye camps, only screening was done by Sai Organization and the patients were taken to regular hospitals for surgery. At Chennai, UDHI Hospital, Voluntary Health Service Hospital, Sundaram Medical Foundation and Sankara Nethralaya collaborated in this activity. Sri. Thyagarajan took an active part at Udhi eye clinic and VHS hospitals.

Cardiac Screening Camp

During 1992, SaiKrupa team organized a Cardiac Screening Camp at Bala Bhavan in T. Nagar. X-ray and ECG with lab support were made available by Swami's grace. Leading cardiologists and radiologists attended this camp. Nearly 400 patients with cardiac problems were screened and those who required cardiac surgery and found fit for the same were referred to Super Speciality Hospital at Puttaparthi. The idea was to reduce the work load of screening at Puttaparthi. During subsequent years this service was replaced by deputing doctors to Puttaparthi for 1 week at a time to assist in screening.

Study Circle and other Spiritual Activities

Work at SaiKrupa begins every Sunday with bhajans for 10 min and before closing, arthi is offered to Bhagawan. During early years, Sri. Rayningar used to conduct Geetha classes exclusively for SaiKrupa team. When Bhagawan introduced Study Circle program, SaiKrupa adopted the same. Dr. Ramsamy, Dr. Venkatramani used to conduct this program for doctors and sevadal volunteers with active participation and discussion. These monthly meetings were organized with unremitting regularity for more than 200 sessions.

Currently, Rudram chanting is done at the beginning of work every Sunday and all patients are served food and drinking water. Annually, gifting of clothes is also done on Bhagawan's birthday to these patients. Notebooks and stationary items are distributed to the students of Anandana Samajam at the beginning of the academic year.

Antony From Anatomy Lab

While I was working as a tutor in operative surgery at Stanley Medical College, it was my duty to do practical demonstration for undergraduate students in the Anatomy dissection hall. It is here that I met Antony – a jovial and happy-go-lucky person. He was a lab assistant and always full of life – he used the term "friends" to refer to skeletons and preserved human bodies in the formalin tank. He would easily identify the body part we had dissected in the previous class, pull it out, wash it, and lay it on the table. He could easily identify the side: right or left of the carpel bones (small bones of the wrist joint) which even seniors in the Anatomy dept. could not do. Somehow he took a liking for me and we became good friends.

Two decades later, I was invited as a guest speaker for the anniversary of Tondiarpet Samithi. They were celebrating it by conducting a service camp at Monegar Choultry (Old Age Home) which was adjacent to Stanley Medical College. There was a common compound wall between Anatomy dept. and Monegar Choultry complex. The devotees had spruced up the entire building and the compound which was most unkempt; they also white washed the walls and water washed the kadappa slab flooring and made the premises spic and span. They provided new clothes – dhothis and angavastram for men, and sarees for ladies. Bhajans were sung and after aarati, hot sweet pongal, and pulihora(Tamarind rice) comprising a sumptuous lunch was served for all inmates. The Sai devotees of Tondiarpet samithi brought the sunshine of Sai love to a place that was gloomy and dreary.

It is while going around and meeting inmates that I found Antony quietly sitting in a corner. He had shrunk to half his original size and all the mirth and dazzle in his eyes were gone. To begin with, he couldn't recognize me. When I called him by name he broke down. He was meeting a friendly face and listening to an affectionate voice after almost a decade since he shifted himself across the compound wall. He informed me that his sons were in USA and Gulf and well off, but had abandoned him. His wife had passed away long ago.

We were talking for almost an hour. He had worn the new clothes and we shared Swami's prasadam. He told me that it was the happiest day of his life and the melodious bhajans had uplifted his dropping spirit and were ringing in his ear long after the bhajans had concluded.

Three hours later, the Samithi convenor called me to inform that Antony went to take a nap on his usual bench and never woke up. Antony had expressed his desire that his body must be handed over to the Anatomy dept., in the adjacent building. A selfless wish to be of use to medical students long after his passing. He died in ecstasy at the "Sai Succor" that reached him, and he happily joined his friends in the formalin tank across the compound.

Bhagawan's Blessings to Doctors

During January 1987, Bhagawan was expected to visit SaiKrupa in the new location. But this did not materialise. He wanted SaiKrupa doctors to come to Abbottsbury. He blessed the ultra short wave therapy equipment – used for Physiotherapy – which was bought for SaiKrupa. He also graciously gifted a stethoscope for each of the assembled doctors. The devotee who had purchased Abbottsbury had prayed to Bhagawan to use the place for His darshan and discourse as usual, since new construction had not yet started at the place. That was the last time Bhagawan visited Abbottsbury.

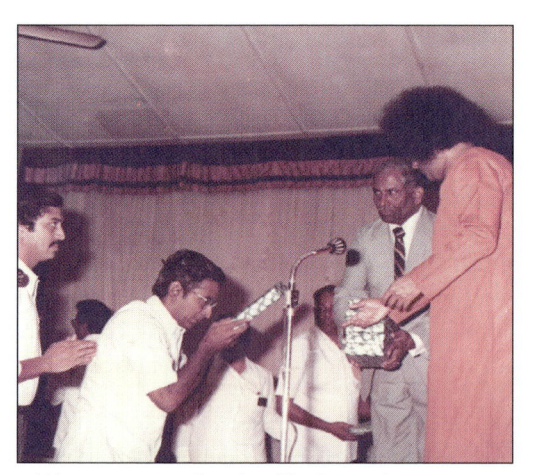

Bhagawan graciously gifted a stethoscope to
each of the assembled doctors

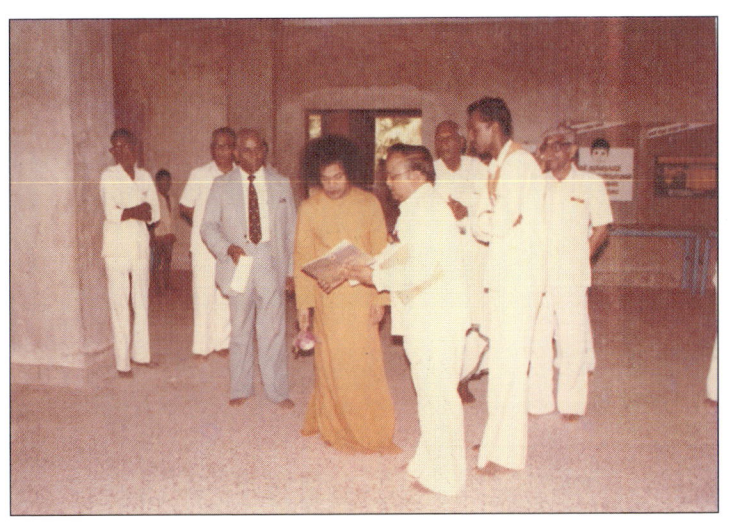

Bhagawan tours new SaiKrupa facility

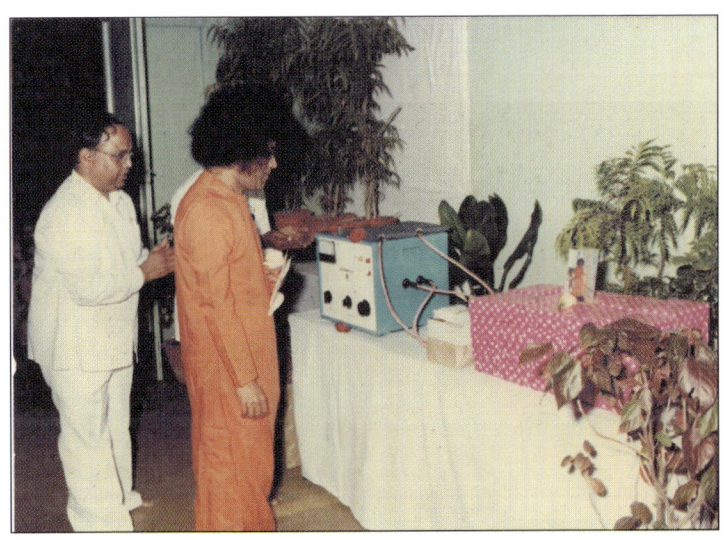

Bhagawan graciously blessed Physiotherapy equipment for SaiKrupa

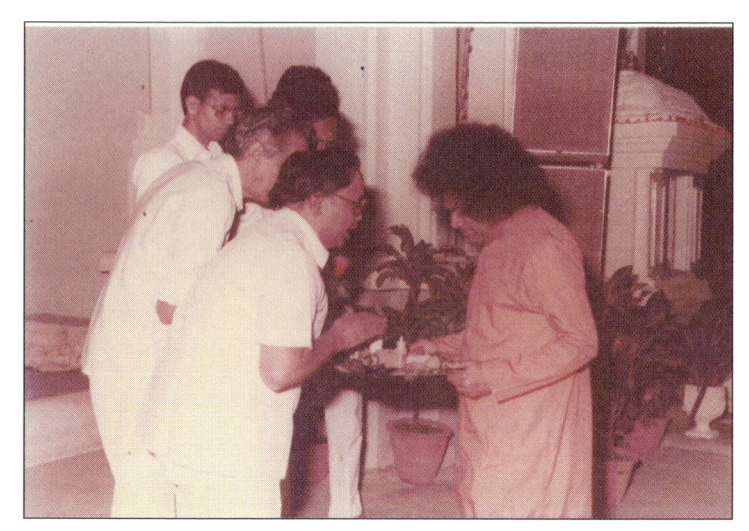

Bhagawan graciously blessed doctors and diagnostic equipment at Sundaram

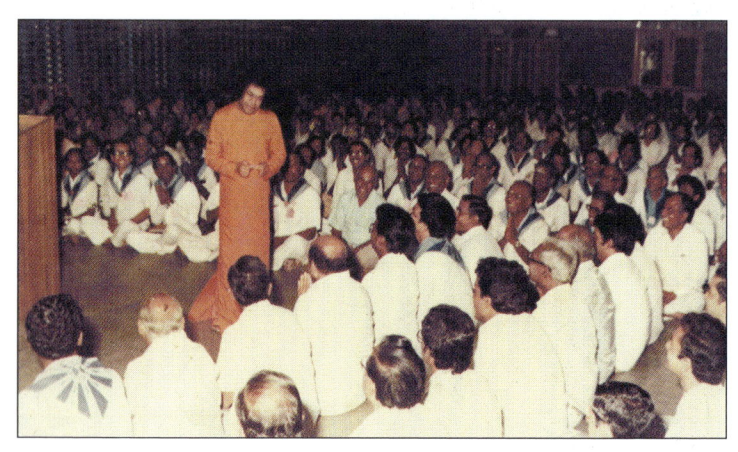

Bhagawan talking to doctors at Abbotsbury, Chennai

Love is Expansion

Under Bhagawan's directions many villages were adopted by Sai Organization, Tamil Nadu. Sevadal were already exposed to service in the domain of Health, by serving in various eye camps. It was felt that training must be imparted to health workers to survey villagers, record health status of local population, and advise them regarding nutrition, personal hygiene, and environmental hygiene.

We contacted various agencies such as UNICEF, Director of Public Health, DANIDA Project, and collected materials – this resulted in preparation of special kits for health workers. A Health workers manual was also printed. I was ably assisted by Sri. M.R. Chandran who was a Director in R.D.L.A. dept. and a sevadal leader. The idea was to give training to 750 sevadals and active workers attending the State Conference at Naradha Gana Sabha Hall, Chennai. (1994). When Bhagawan's Blessings were sought, His reaction was "Why only 750? Why not all 900 delegates attending the Conference?" Love is expansion; His directions and Love enabled us to equip adequate kits and exhibition materials for the additional number. Swami was very happy with the planned arrangements. He even deputed His Vice Chancellor Sri. Sampath to preside over the inauguration. Sri. Sampath stayed on for the full program and remarked that a new dimension to further Bhagawan's mission had been made visible.

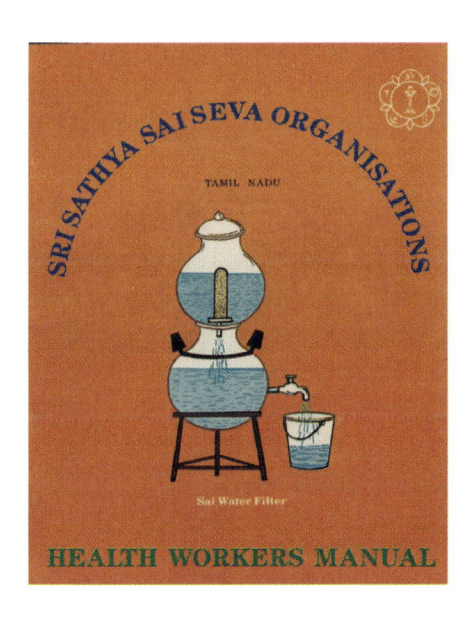

Medical Seva at Prashanthi & Whitefield

O.P. Service at Prashanthi Nilayam and Whitefield

To augment and assist in the O.P. work of screening cardiac patients, devotee doctors were deputed to Prashanthi Nilayam. Dr. T. Ram Manohar Rao was appointed as National Coordinator for this activity. From SaiKrupa, a father and son duo – Dr. Padmanaban and Dr. Vijayaraghavan – both physicians and professors of medicine, regularly attended this one week service at Prashanthi Nilayam. Subsequently this facility was extended to the General Hospital at Puttaparthi as well as at Whitefield. I had the blessed opportunity to serve at Whitefield General Hospital for two weeks.

During Bhagawan's Birthday(every year), medical camps were organized to provide immediate medical aid to devotees for a period of about a week. Dr. Rama Devi, Dr. Lakshmi Devi, Dr. Manimegalai, Dr. Sujaya, Dr. Monica and Dr. Prathiba regularly offered their services for a week during this period along with others. Dr. Thangavelu and Dr. Radhakrishnan - Ophthalmologists from Coimbatore were other members who used to offer full-time service for this camp as well as General Hospital duties.

International Medical Conference at Prashanthi Nilayam – 2005

Dr. T. Ram Manohar Rao, Dr. Sundaram, Dr. Lakshminarayana, Dr. Rama Devi, Dr. Lakshmi Devi, Dr. Kumari Menon, and myself represented SaiKrupa at the International Medical Conference. I was entrusted with the task of organizing Indian Section of the International Exhibition on medical seva. Bhagawan visited the exhibition and blessed everyone.

Mother and Child Program at Prashanthi Nilayam (from 2007)

Dr. Kumari Menon and Dr. Geetha from Saikrupa, used to visit Prashanthi Nilayam every month from 19th for a week and participate in this Mother and Child Program by going around villages along with the mobile hospital unit. They have assisted in promoting hospital delivery, immunization and child care, preparing a unique dossier for every child - complete with immunization history for a period of five years from birth - in the area covered by this scheme. This is an ongoing service, which is currently in its 10th year of operation.

Visiting Consultants from SaiKrupa

Dr. Mohan Kumaresh, Oncologist – and Dr. V. Mohan, – diabetologist have been regularly visiting Prashanthi Nilayam hospitals as consultants. Prof. S. Ramaswamy visits as a faculty in anatomy for the Post Graduates at Sri

Sathya Institute of Higher Medical Sciences. Dr. Sundarajan, Plastic Surgeon, and Mrs. Kalyani Sundarajan, from Anna Nagar SaiKrupa have been visiting General Hospitals at Puttaparthi and Whitefield as consultants, every month. Dr. Hiramalini and Dr. Seshadri Harihar have been visiting both the General Hospitals every month as consultants in Rheumatology and Psychiatry respectively. Dr. Rama Devi, Dr. Laksmi Devi and Dr. Girija Devi offer their services at Puttaparthi General Hospital whenever they visit Puttaparthi.

> "The food that you consume must have two important qualities for it to provide proper nourishment to the body. It must have been 1) Dharmarjitham - earned out of righteous means; 2) Daivarpitham - consecrated to God before partaking of it."
>
> Divide your stomach into 4 parts. Fill two parts with satwick food. Fill one part with water. And leave the rest for air. This is the correct proportion for proper digestion and assimilation. Avoid stale food. Always eat freshly cooked food. It's a good habit to starve once in 15 days atleast."- Baba

Health Meters for Auto Drivers

Auto rickshaws are small three wheelers which can carry two passengers and easily negotiate the congested streets and bylanes of the city of Chennai. They are said to be omnipresent – more than 50,000 plying in the city roads. Some of the drivers are a law unto themselves and are prone to traffic accidents. They are also the first responders in the event of a road side emergency, transporting patients to nearby hospitals.

General health awareness is very low for this group - health screening or regular check up is almost absent. Hence it was decided to do a thorough health screening for this group.

A simple survey was conducted among these unorganized groups. Their health awareness was very poor and a good percentage were given to smoking and addicted to alcohol. None were covered by health insurance, and many plying owned vehicles were not covered for accidents. Health screening and regular check up was totally absent.

A special ID was designed with all particulars, photograph, blood group, and known risk factors regarding health and record of medication they were on, and their physician contact numbers.

Routine B.P., blood sugar, blood grouping, and vision testing were done for all. Those requiring corrective lens were provided prescription glasses. Dr. V. Mohan and his team provided free life time treatment for those diagnosed with diabetes at his hospital.

All Auto Drivers were taught basic First Aid and especially C.P.R.(Cardio Pulmonary Resuscitation) using a Mannequin provided by Anesthesia Foundation. Dr. Sarawathi was in charge of this task. Auto Drivers were educated about nutrition and the evils of drinking and smoking. Gradually, this brought about a transformation in their habits and life style.

Many such screening cum training camps were conducted at different areas by different cluster of Sai centers for a period of little over a year covering nearly 20% of this section of society. Services were offered in a atmosphere of spiritual vibrations and continuous bhajan singing. This brought about a great change in their attitude and behavior. Many Drivers started emulating Sevadals and some came and offered seva at subsequent camps. This is the beneficial effect of good company. Bhagawan has said many a time: "Tell me your company and I shall tell who you are."

Some Drivers informed us of having visited Prashanthi Nilayam along with their families and were blessed to have Bhagawan's darshan. Seeing our youth sevadal volunteers many gave up smoking, alchohol, and non-vegetarian food. Some Drivers reported to SaiKrupa for service and on their way back offered free rides to patients upto the bus stand; many drivers started attending bhajans at Sundaram and joined as members of Samithi.

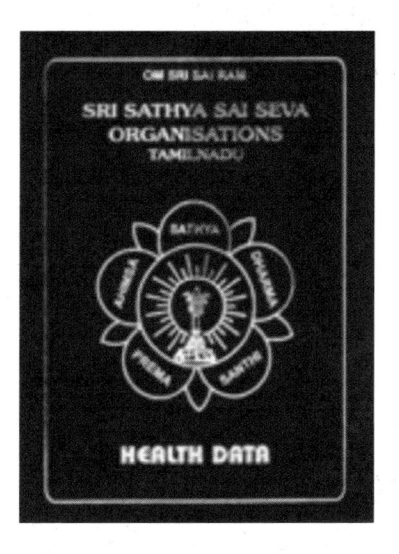

Passport size health data book for auto drivers, used for follow up care

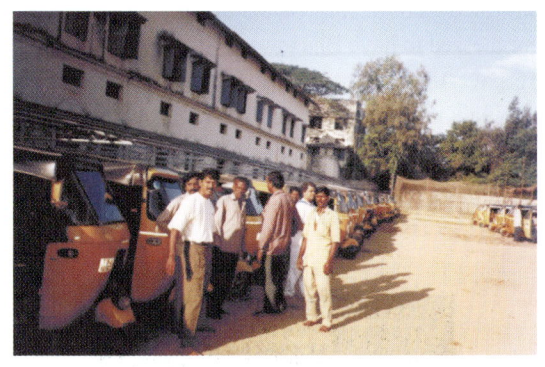

Autos parked in an orderly manner at camp site, organized by Sevadals

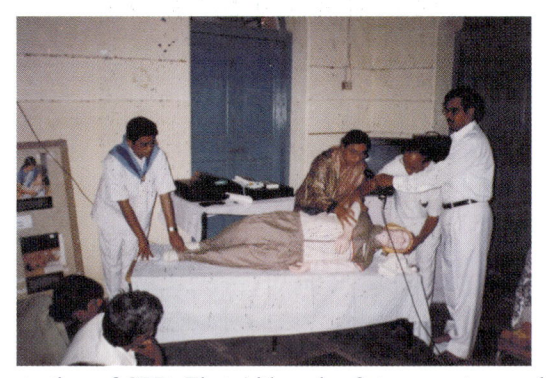

Demonstration of CPR, First Aid, and safe transport procedures to Auto Drivers with the aid of a mannequin.

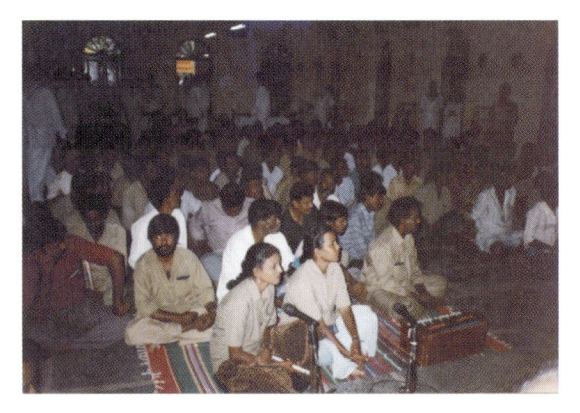

Auto Drivers listening in rapt attention to CPR demonstation

Humanising Medicare

Apart from regular training classes and updates for our health workers, SaiKrupa has organized seminars and symposia for the medical fraternity in the city of Chennai.

A seminar on **"Humanising Medicare"** was conducted at Triple Helix auditorium in CLRI campus on 9th March 2003. Smt. Girija Vaidyanathan, IAS, Secretary dept of health and family welfare – Govt. of Tamil Nadu – lighted the lamp of love and gave the inaugural address. Sri. G.K. Raman, Trust Convenor, welcomed the gathering and Sri. V. Srinivasan, All India President, delivered the keynote address. Prof. K.V. Thiruvenkatam, Senior Prof. of Medicine, who was the chief guest, highlighted on ethics in medical practices. There was a special address by Sri. Vijaya Krishnan – Alumnus of Sri Sathya Sai Institute of Higher Learning.

The highlight of the entire program was the star studded panel discussion on Human Values, with Prof. N. Rangabhasyam, senior surgical gastroenterologist acting as a moderator.

Prof. U. Mohamed, physician and diabetologist expounded on the value of "Truth" in medical practice, extensively quoting from the Koran.

Prof. S. S. Badrinath, vitreo-retinal surgeon, highlighted the value of "Right Conduct" and empathy in medical practice.

Prof. Matangi Ramakrishnan, plastic and reconstructive surgeon, highlighted the value of "Peace" and the right approach to a patient's problem.

Prof. Pritika Chary, neuro physician and neurosurgeon, talked on the value of "Love" in the management of patients and how to elicit maximum compliance from a patient.

Prof. P.V. Chandrashekaran, cardiologist, propounded on the value of "Non-Violence" and positive approach in handling a patient.

That such a galaxy of experts and specialists were able to meet and discuss not only medical topics but also on ethics and values was sheer Sai grace. Over 350 doctors and specialists were awe struck and grateful for such a unique experience and an intellectual treat. There was lively 30 min audience participation.

The icing on the cake was the skit enacted by the tiny tots of Sri Sathya Sai Balavikas entitled "The Importance of Character". With this, the program came to an end.

Sri Sathya Sai Healthcare Project(2007)

Bhagawan graciously permitted Tamil Nadu, and Chennai in particular, the coveted opportunity to conduct Athi Rudra Maha Yagnam in His immediate divine presence during Jan. 2007. A special 10 acre site was converted into a "Yagnashala"(sacred site for performance of vedic rituals) with full infrastructure – roads, residential buildings, dining halls, kitchen and a brand new bungalow for Bhagawan's stay were all constructed at Tiruvanmiyur. This massive function with devotees from all over the globe was a sight for Gods to see. SaiKrupa was given the opportunity to provide medical care for the visiting devotees, rithwiks (priests who perform vedic rituals) and volunteers.

One of the major events during Athi Rudra Maha Yagna was the inauguration of Sri Sathya Sai Health Care Project by Bhagawan. Nearly 80 institutions from Chennai including hospitals, nursing homes, laboratories, diagnostic clinics, etc. offered their services and willingness to spare one bed for free medical service.

When Sai Organization started working out the details of the 10 day program in connection with Ati Rudra Maha Yagnam, it was planned to have cultural programs each evening and the famous artist and musicians who are Bhagawan's devotees would be given a chance to perform in the divine presence. An idea was also mooted to have special darshan each evening for a invited group, with reserved seating arrangement. A day was allotted for IAS(Indian Administrative Service) officers, bureaucrats and heads of govt. institutions. One evening, it was industrialists and leading businessmen. In this manner, an evening got allotted for leading medical professionals; lawyers and judges an evening; and engineers and technocrats on another evening.

For the evening reserved for medical professionals, Dr. T. Ram Manohar Rao, Dr. E. Prabhu, Sri. N. Ramani, and Prof. Dr. N. Rangabhashyam (leading surgical gastro enterologist) met and chalked out the details. During this meeting, the idea was mooted to pledge one bed free, in the service of patients referred by Sai Organization. This would be as a response to Bhagawan's request to doctors to spare few hours a week in providing care for those who cannot afford to pay, as a 'free service'(Divine Discourse: Valedictory function, International Cardiology Conference, SSSIHMS, Puttaparthi). By word of mouth, the news spread like wild fire, and within 48 hours, 80 institutions gave their willingness to join the project. These included not only hospitals and nursing homes but also a nuclear lab, several diagnostic and pathology labs, and x-ray clinics.

Already, this kind of service was being undertaken by Kumaran Hospitals, VHS Hospital, Shankar Netralaya, and Sundaram Medical Foundation, and Madras ENT Research Institute. A nursing home in Anna Nagar(Sri Devi Hospital) had Sri Sathya Sai ward with 4 beds committed for free service. Bhagawan inaugurated SSS Healthcare project and blessed the networking institutions by presenting a health kit each. Prof. N. Rangabhashyam spoke on behalf of all members and expressed gratitude for the opportunity for service provided by Bhagawan and for His benediction. Subsequently, Radiosai did a full story on the project and hailed it as a Virtual Super Speciality Hospital.

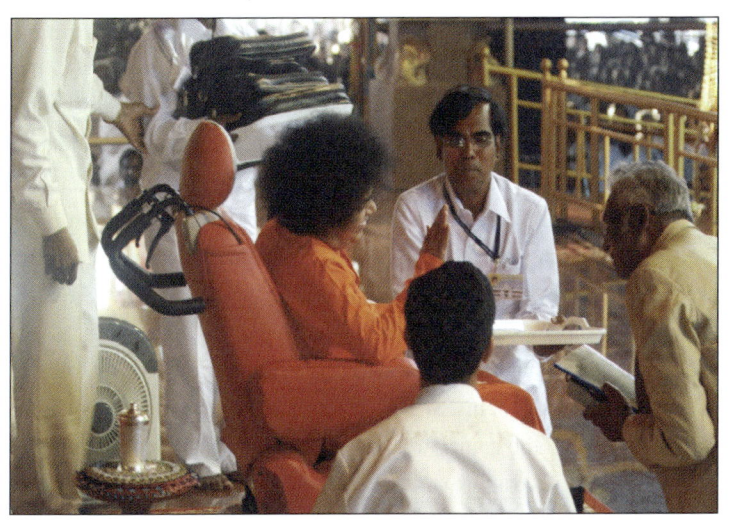

Bhagawan graciously blessing Dr. Rangabhasyam who addressed the gathering on behalf of private institutions participating in Sathya Sai Healthcare project

Sri Sathya Sai Total Healthcare – A Working Model

The campus of Sri Ramachandra Medical College (Chennai), its massive air conditioned auditorium, and its environs were converted in to a mini Prashanthi Nilayam – with arches, festoons, large flex prints of 20' x 12' of both the super specialty hospitals. There was a large backdrop on the stage with Bhagawan's picture and the title of the symposium. The CCTV with multiple videoscope screens gave a close and detailed perspective of the proceedings.

The symposium on "Sri Sathya Sai Total Health Care – a working model" was conducted on 17th July 2010 and was formally inaugurated by the lighting of the lamp of love by Sri. Venkatachalam – pro chancellor of SRM University. Bhagawan had deputed Dr. Safaya, Director of Sathya Sai Super Speciality Hospital, Prashanthigram to deliver the keynote address. The union deputy minister of health and family welfare was the chief guest. Dr. Krishna Raman, convenor of SaiKrupa welcomed the gathering. Prof. K. V. Thiruvengadam addressed the gathering and lauded the Sai organization for its philanthropic approach to medical seva. Dr. Safaya traced the history of Sri Sathya Sai Institute of Higher Medical Sciences and how Bhagawan made the impossible possible and offered a world class tertiary medical care in a remote rural setting, totally free of cost to anyone seeking help. Sri. V. Srinivasan, All India President of Sai Organization was on the panel answering queries and clearing doubts from audience which numbered approximately 600 doctors and medical students.

SaiKrupa Events

On completion of the first year of seva at SaiKrupa, all of us – doctors, paramedics, and sevadal – joined and went on a overnight trip by a chartered bus to Parthi(May 1, 1980 – it was a holiday due to labour day). During morning darshan, Bhagawan blessed us by signing in the SaiKrupa register. We were in ecstasy at Bhagawan's compassion. We boarded the bus in the evening for overnight return trip. We were blissfully ignorant of the convention that we had to seek Bhagawan's permission before leaving Parthi.

But the merciful Lord sent a hamper full of vibhuti packets to the bus, with a message that He had planned to give padanamaskar the following morning and since we had already boarded the bus, He was sending prasadam. We realized our mistake and on reaching Madras, we wrote a letter of gratitude to the compassionate Lord.

Bhagawan gives a new role to play

It was 1986, an entirely new Sathya Sai Trust was nominated for Tamil Nadu. I was overwhelmed when I learnt that Bhagawan had nominated me as one of the 5 members of Sathya Sai Trust (Tamil Nadu). All of us went to Whitefield for His darshan after we took charge. Bhagawan was full of love and like a mother gave detailed instructions and guidance and blessed us all to function like the five fingers of the hand.

Because of the rule that no person should hold 2 different posts, I was obliged to relinquish my post as the convener of the medical unit and SaiKrupa. But I am continuing as a volunteer doctor and do not miss my Sunday seva at SaiKrupa as long as I am in station.

Currently, Dr. E. Prabhu is the overall in-charge of medical seva in Tamil Nadu. Sri.Kanakaraj and Sri. Mahendran manage the day-to-day affairs of main SaiKrupa. By Bhagawan's grace, there are 11 SaiKrupa clinics conducting medical seva in Tamil Nadu.

10th Anniversary

On Easwaramma Day 1989 - A decade of medical seva was celebrated at Sundaram. Sri. Arjuna Raja, trust convenor was the chief guest. Sri. Kandasamy – another senior trust member also participated. All doctors who had been with us from day one, Sri. Sankara Subramanium who had been like a manager looking after administrative work, postings, drug purchase, accounts, etc. – were honoured.

Momentos were distributed to all members.

25th Anniversary

After completion of 25 years, we had a grand function, this time at Chennapuri Anadana Samajam, where Saikrupa is functioning. The function was arranged in the beautifully decorated upstairs hall. Sri. G.K. Raman, then trust convener, was the chief guest. Dr. Kumari Menon made a presentation on the growth of Saikrupa for a quarter century. One of the volunteers prepared a silver coin to commemorate the occasion.

36th Anniversary and Gratitude Program

As a part of Bhagawan's 90th birthday celebrations, we had a "SaiKrupa gratitude program" expressing our gratitude to Bhagawan for completing 36 years in His service. Dr. V. Mohan who is a member of SaiKrupa and also our trust convener presided over the function. We had a symposium on "Transformation through medical seva". The function which was arranged in the main hall of Sundaram was attended by more than 300 doctors from all over Tamil Nadu and the Sevadal members who serve at various SaiKrupa locations. Sri. V. Srinivasan, All India President, delivered the keynote address "Medical Seva – the way forward".

SaiKrupa Doctors Serving Global Human Family

Many SaiKrupa doctors have distinguished themselves through service in their respective specialities. It has been said that it is impossible to escape self impact when serving and God cares much more for what one becomes through service than the service itself. Service is an opportunity, a means to an end; the end being self transformation.

Many doctors who served at SaiKrupa in Chennai are currently spread across India and the globe - serving in many prestigious and consequential roles, delivering medical care suffused with Sai ideals to the global human family. The import of Bhagawan's aphorism that there is only one caste - the caste of humanity - has become a part of our experience. In a subtle but profound way...Bhagawan has architected the spread of His ideals through young doctors who served at SaiKrupa. One cannot help but marvel at Bhagawan's expansive vision for uplifting humanity. That He gave us a chance to play a role in this divine mission overwhelms us with gratitude.

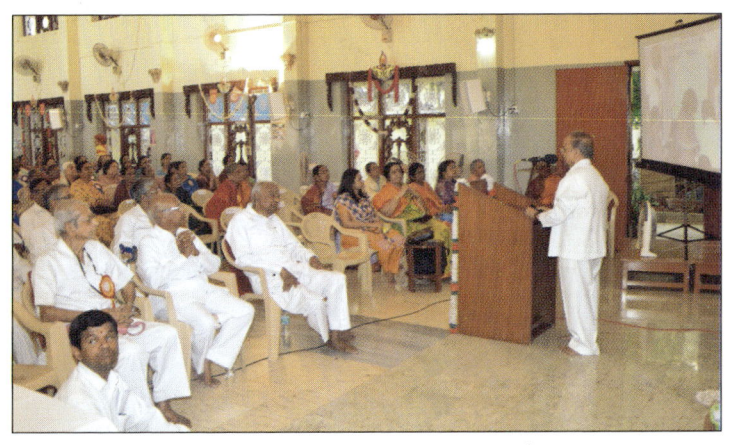

Gratitude program at Sundaram to mark the 36th anniversary of SaiKrupa which coincided with 90th year of advent of Bhagawan Sri Sathya Sai Baba, Aug. 2015

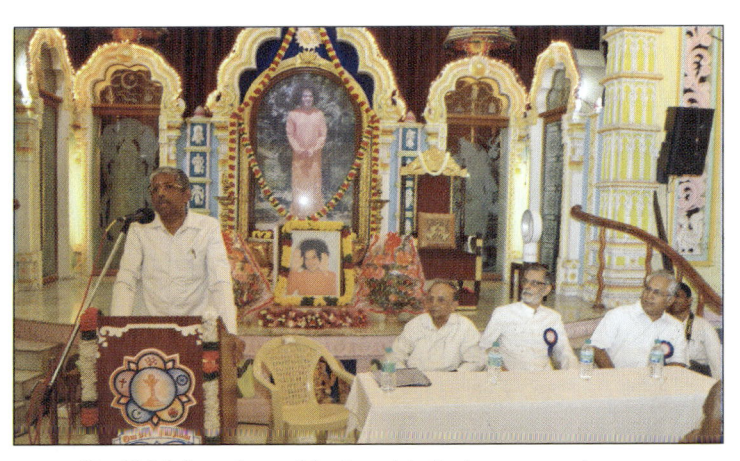

Dr. V. Mohan shares his thoughts during symposium on transformation through medical seva

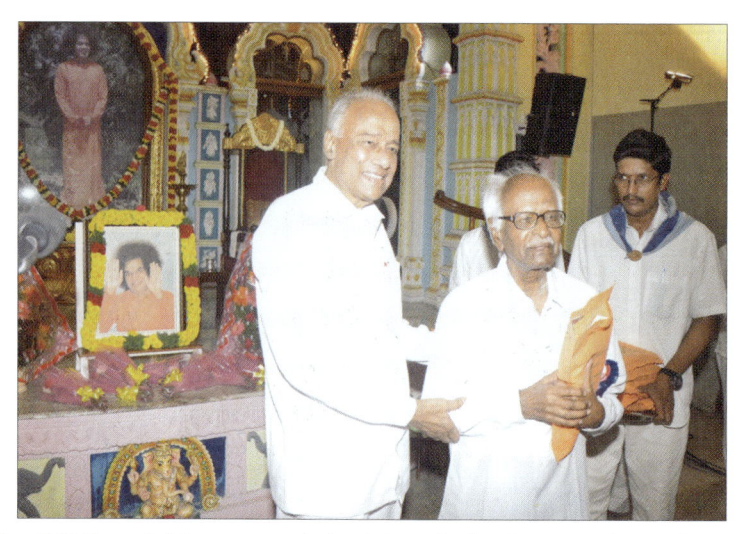

Dr. G.V. Ramakrishna, general physician who has been serving patients at SaiKrupa since the days of inception being felicitated by Sri. V. Srinivasan, then All India President of Sai Organization, during event held to commemorate 36th anniversary of SaiKrupa, Aug. 2015

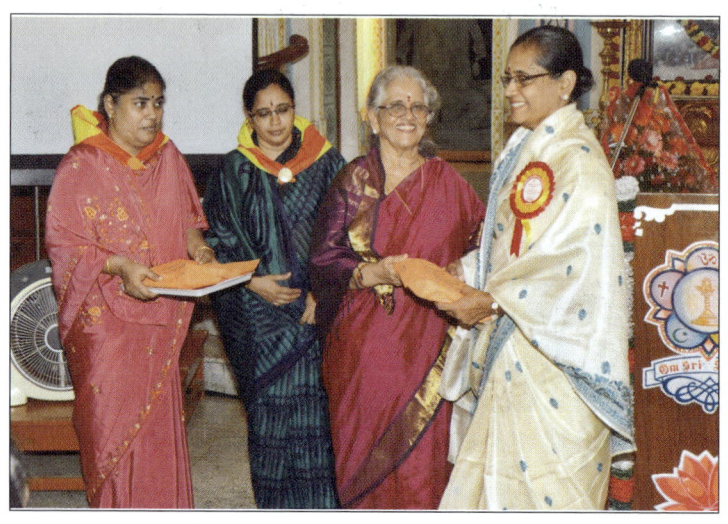

Dr. Kumari Menon, long serving pediatrician at SaiKrupa being felicitated by Mrs. Vidya Srinivasan, National Coordinator for Balvikas, at the 36th anniversary of SaiKrupa, Aug. 2015

Section 3 –

Personal Experiences

First Encounter: Earliest Prescriptions

Just before dasara celebrations, 1967, we visited Parthi for the first time. We had travelled for nearly 23 hours before, by different modes of transport, including a bullock cart and by foot on the dry river bed of Chitravathi. Just then, Bhagawan had finished his supper and was walking back to His room on the verandah of the first floor of Prashanthi mandir. That was the last darshan for the day and nearly 50 people were waiting in the compound to have a glimpse of Baba and we joined them, having just unloaded our luggage from the bullock cart. As we were entering the compound, Bhagawan was about to enter His room, turned to our side, giving us a glimpse before disappearing into His chamber.

We were directed towards a large tin roofed shed with sandy floor, for resting for the night. We were too tired to even think of food. We spread the bed sheets we had brought and hit the sandy bed, so to say. We were about 60 people occupying the shed for the night. Having come to know that there are no wash room facilities, and in the cover of early morning darkness, we had to complete ablutions in the open field, my father(who had been a city bird) declared: the place is God forsaken and we should quit first thing in the morning.

By about 4:00 a.m. next morning, a tall gentleman with a long torch light approached us enquiring where was the judge who has come from Trichy. I took him to my father. He announced that his name was Suraiah and that Baba had allotted a room for us in the first floor of Vedapatashala. He handed over the keys and directed us to go behind the mandir to reach the place allotted. We packed our things and headed to the room allotted. My father was amply relieved to find the room had a toilet attached(Indian style). The cement around the closet had not yet dried and there was a small tap and a bucket.

We went to Chitravathi river side to the makeshift bathing cubicles where hot water was available for 4 annas(25 paise) a kodum (metal pot for storing water).

By about 9:00 a.m., we were ready and leisurely planning to visit the mandir where bhajan singing was going on. Lo and behold, we found Baba walking up the steps towards the verandah opposite our room where we were standing. We were dumbfounded. Baba walked up to us and holding the grill on one side, started conversing with the lorry driver who was unloading construction jelly in front of the building. Baba enquired from the driver as to the cause of his late arrival, when he was actually expected the previous night. The driver was explaining how he was held up at the check post. Baba commented saying why he did not pay him "mamool" of Rs. 2 at the counter. Smiling, He turned towards us saying "we should not talk such things before a judge?"

We had not announced to anybody who we are and where from we had arrived. Our decision to go to Parthi was 11th hour decision. Here was Baba, who had not only allotted a room at 4:00 a.m. but also talking about us to a 3rd person! He enquired about our comfort and conversed with such a familiar, friendly, and disarming manner. He talked about everything – weather, politics, new govt. at Madras(C.N. Annadurai had formed the first non-congress govt. in Tamil Nadu), etc. And, enough personal details about each of us to indicate how intimately He knows us. We were so awestruck that we did not even ask Him to come inside the very room He had so generously allotted. It was well over 1 hour, and Sri. Kasturi had come up to the steps twice already to indicate that Aarti time was up.

"I think I have charged your batteries enough for today, I'll come again tomorrow!" so declaring, He proceeded downstairs towards the mandir.

We had no concept of an interview and how valuable it was to have Baba talking to us for 1 hour.

We spruced up the room, swept and swabbed. We borrowed a wooden chair from a neighbour and spread a silk saree on it. My wife was ready with a palmyra leaf (Phunkah) she had purchased for fanning. There was no fan or power connection to the room.

As promised, Baba arrived the following morning by about 9:00 a.m. He left His foot wear outside before entering and sat on the chair. He asked all of us to sit comfortably. I informed Him about how my father had slipped and fallen down near the bathing cubicle and sustained a fracture in his leg. And that he was in great pain. Baba waved His hand, and materialized vibhuthi, and gave to my father to be swallowed immediately. Baba asked him to stretch both legs and sit comfortably. Baba assured me that it was not a fracture but the leg had got twisted. There was immediate pain relief and he was comfortable enough to ask a few questions to Baba.

But I was not mentally happy. Here I was, a medical officer, working in the casualty dept. of a teaching hospital, where I daily attend atleast on a dozen road accident cases with multiple fractures. I found my father having a swelling on fall, a typically crackling on touch, and extreme pain. How can it not be a fracture? I took Baba's diagnosis with a pinch of salt.

In the meanwhile, Baba had invited some spiritual questions and my father was ready with a barrage of them. I recollect a couple of them now even after half a century has passed by.

1. Why good people always have problems and miseries. While obviously, evil doers are leading a comfortable life enjoying all luxuries?

Baba explained saying: if you sow ragi, you will be consuming the same after harvest during the next season, though you may be sowing paddy at that time. A person who had harvested Paddy will be consuming the same, though currently he may be sowing ragi.

What you go through in life is the result and reaction of your past karma.

This led my father to ask the 2nd question: why do innocent children suddenly die at a tender age when they have not had a chance to do bad karma?

Baba cited the example of one buying a new cloth from a reduction sale and stitching a pant and the same getting torn the very first time it is worn. Baba explained saying, "for you it may be a new pant, but for the shop keeper, it was an old stock for clearance sale. As soon as the past karma is redeemed, the soul returns to the source."

The explanations were so down-to-earth and easy to understand. That is the uniqueness of Swami.

Baba wanted us to stay for 10 days and participate in the Dassara festivities which were imminent. We pleaded our inability because both myself and my father were govt. servants and cannot take long leave. We then took leave of Baba. Swami returned to the mandir after having spent 1 hour with us and sent prasadam packets through Sri. N. Kasturi.

On our return journey, we halted at Bangalore and had an x-ray done for my father. I was shocked to find a "torsion fracture of fibula"! –this is described as "drumstick fracture" even in medical text books. If a drum stick, a vegetable called murrungaikai in Tamil, is twisted forcibily, it breaks inside but remains intact without shattering into pieces because of the outer sheath. Of all the 300 odd bones in the body, this type of fracture can occur only in the fibula – a bone supporting calf muscles! How accurate was Bhagawan's diagnosis!

Our respect and awe for Swami started growing from that moment and has not stopped.

It sounds incredible that Swami came walking to our room and talked to us on two consecutive days for an hour on each occasion. I realized the importance of the invaluable gift of divine time during the subsequent visits, many of which, I had to spend the nights under the canopy of stars. I had to wait 18 long years and many dozens of trips to Parthi before I had a chance for the coveted interview in Swami's room. Even then, it was Bhagawan who gave an explanation for the long interval. He said, "each time you have been coming with Chunnilal, stay for a day and run away. This is the first time, you have come with your family. Should I not meet them? That is why I called you in."

Bhagawan's love is unfathomable. We were deeply touched by the warmth of His affection. He knows every detail about each of us, not only in this life time, but since time began, during which we have been following Him. That should be enough incentive to long to merge back into Him.

Dr. Sitaramiah was already 77 years old and had a long innings of serving at Puttaparthi General Hospital -very often as a lone medical officer – pleaded with Bhagawan to be relived of the responsibility. Swami brushed aside his protestations and encouraged him to continue as enthusiastically as hitherto saying:

"Do not be afraid. Be but an instrument. I will do everything for you." - Baba

Cases Referred by Bhagawan

Medical care, especially secondary and tertiary care is built on referrals from primary care and other specialists. This is how healthcare system is organized in most countries. It is an honour to be referred cases … often it is a sign of peer recognition of skills a practioner has developed. It is a blessing when Bhagawan Himself, the doctor of doctors, refers cases. In this case, it is a sign of grace than of mere professional competence; for the Lord had decided to use us as His instruments.

I digress here to recall the story of Dr. Upadhya, an Ophthalmic surgeon from U.K. Dr. Upadhya had returned from an eye camp in Pune, where they had run out of supplies of medicine and had given lower dosage. Swami didn't approve the reduction of dosage due to lack of supply. Dr. Upadhya humbly asked Swami what is to be done in cases where there is no recourse to proper treatment due to lack of supply or other reasons. Swami then asked, what do you do when you have to refer a case to another specialist. Dr. Upadhya replied saying "Swami, I write a referral note to the specialist". Then Swami said, "give the patient Vibhuti. That is your referral note to me. I'll take care of the patient." This interaction reveals to the world that He is the doctor of doctors and Vibhuti is the referral note to the divine specialist.

Digression complete, let me return back to instances where Bhagawan referred cases to SaiKrupa.

Implant to restore hearing

Bhagawan deputed the postmaster at Parthi saying "take your daughter to Madras. Our doctors at Abbotsbury will attend on her and she will be alright." It was a privilege and blessing for SaiKrupa to attend on her. Dr. Selvanarayanan, ENT surgeon operated on her ear, using an imported microscope and a Teflon implant, in his own nursing home to restore her hearing. He not only offered his service and facilities free of cost but also provided an extra room for her parents to stay during the period of treatment.

Undiagnosed fever

I heard Bhagawan calling "doctor, doctor" from the inner interview room where Swami had taken a family for a private audience. I was sitting in the outer common interview room along with others, and was not sure whether the call was meant for me. The head of the family who had gone in along with Swami, came out and beckoned saying "Swami is calling you." When both entered the inner room,

Swami made fun of us saying "Both are doctors, sitting side by side, without knowing each other until this doctor called you in." Swami paused and asked "Who is a better doctor you or I?" Bhagawan introduced the family and wanted to know from me as to who was the best gastroenterologist at Madras. He wanted me to take the other doctor's son who was studying in Swami's school, to Madras, and show him to the best physician and specialist, and have him treated for his jaundice which had not responded to any treatment available at Parthi.

The patient was personally taken to Prof. K.M. Lakshminarayanan, a physician of repute, for primary consultation and organizing investigations. On eliciting a detailed history, the doctor arrived at the fact that few newly born calves - at the farm house of the patient's grandfather in the village where he had spent his vacation - had died one after another in a strange manner. This boy had played with those calves. The physician felt that it could be a rare case of Brucellosis - a cattle disease affecting human contacts. To clinch the diagnosis the physician ordered a "Rosewald's test" to be done. Unfortunately none of the labs in the city offered this test.

Another Dr. Lakshminarayana (Director, Institute of Microbiology, Madras Medical College) came to my rescue. He offered to run the test in his lab. The test proved positive. This confirmed the diagnosis. He also ran a test on antibiotic sensitivity. Strangely, the sample was resistant to all higher antibiotics but susceptible to Sulpha. No doubt all the antibiotics prescribed at Parthi were ineffective. A course of Sulphadiazine tablets from SaiKrupa found the patient on the road to recovery.

Bhagawan had given a cover containing Rs. 5,000 to the father of the patient to cover for the treatment at Madras, and he was able to return the same to Swami as the tests and treatment did not cost any money.

Retinal Detachment

SaiKrupa was also privileged to give supportive service to a patient referred by Bhagawan to Sankar Netralaya for treatment of retinal detachment.

Conversing with her and her husband, I learned about the depth of their devotion and the manifold love and grace showered on them by Bhagawan. The couple had only two sons. Both of them passed away while studying in Swami's college. The first one passed away due to a medical condition. And within a short time the second boy also died because of a tragic road accident. That the mother could narrate their story calmly as though it was a third person shows the fortitude she had built because of Bhagawan and how much of the void was filled with Swami's love. Both of them are still residents of the ashram in Parthi, in their 70's, fully active in Bhagawan's seva.

Illness cured

Swami called Sri. Rao a senior official of the central Trust, handed him two air tickets to Madras and informed that He will be sending His car the following morning for Mr. Rao and his wife to be dropped at Bangalore airport. Swami's advice was to go to Madras and have treatment for his condition. He asked him not to carry any reports done at Parthi. He wanted him to have all investigations done fresh.

Mr. Rao was pleasantly surprised to find a reception team at Madras airport, consisting of state president, Maj. Gen. S.P. Mahadevan; state Sevadal convenor Sri. N. Ramani, and myself on behalf of SaiKrupa. On Bhagawan's instructions 48 hours prior, arrangements were ready to admit Mr. Rao into Apollo hospital.

Mr. Rao was suffering from chronic stomach pain, loss of appetite, and inability to retain solid food. He was on semi solid and liquid diet and had lost considerable weight.

All the preliminary tests and x-rays were done. Dr. Chakravarthy, the consulting surgeon was of the opinion that Mr. Rao was having a obstructive pathology and wanted to do a window laparotomy and if possible, to bypass the obstruction via short circuiting procedure. Laproscopy had not yet been introduced at that time.

Mr. Rao's nephew was studying in Swami's college. Bhagawan granted him special leave for one month and sent him to Madras to assist Mrs. Rao and provide personal care to Mr. Rao. Mr. and Mrs. Rao did not have children of their own. Bhagawan also deputed Col. Joga Rao - a central Trust member - for a couple of days during surgery to provide moral support.

Permission was obtained from Bhagawan for surgery and the same was proceeded with. Being an Anesthesiologist, I was permitted to be in the operating room during surgery. On opening the abdomen, they found the intestines, stomach, liver, etc., were plastered together. The cancerous growth from the stomach had spread all over. The surgeon had no way of doing any procedure. He expressed his anguish, took a small bit of tissue as biopsy for pathological diagnosis and for a possible chemo therapy.

The surgeon himself wrote a letter addressed to Swami about his findings and likely poor outcome and advised chemo therapy.

Dr. Chakravarthy, myself, and others were very skeptical. The removal of sutures were staggered to 10th and 12th days fearing a bust abdomen. But the recovery was uneventful. On the advice of Bhagawan, Mr. Rao was shifted to St. Isabel's hospital for recuperating. Dr. Chakravarthy agreed to visit him at that hospital also.

Mr. Rao started recovering and retaining semi solid food. The IV drips were discontinued. He started to regain his health and put on some weight. Within 2 weeks of surgery, Mr. Rao was walking down to the hospital canteen for his breakfast. Everybody was amazed to find him gulping down the massive idly(south Indian breakfast delicacy made of rice and lentils) with ease.

Mr. Rao was a workaholic and started attending to and corresponding on Trust matters.

By the 4th week, he wanted me to arrange for permission to leave the hospital for a couple of hours to consult the Trust lawyer who was at Madras. Though I offered to arrange to bring the lawyer to his room, he refused saying "its not proper etiquette." The lawyer was surprised to find Mr. Rao climbing up to his chamber on 1st floor, hardly a month after surgery.

Mr. Rao was discharged after the first course of chemo therapy. He was able to walk up to the aircraft, carrying his own shoulder bag on his way back to Parthi.

He reported for second dose of chemo therapy after a month having regained his original health. Bhagawan advised him to stop chemo therapy after the second dose. I could not meet Mr. Rao subsequently and how the end came is described beautifully in Sathyam Shivam Sundaram, vol. 6.

It was a great learning experience for me: I realized the limitation of medical science and the limitless power of God's love.

Lower Jaw Reconstruction

An MBA student was referred by Bhagawan... He had a tumor in his lower jaw. Fortunately, the biopsy proved that it was non-malignant; but, the left half of the lower jaw had to be removed. We had him admitted in a private nursing home. The plastic surgeon was able to do a neat job and there was no disfigurement and the scar hardly visible. On seeing his profile, nobody could say that his lower jaw(left half) was missing. On seeing the loving care provided by SaiKrupa doctors and the sevadals visiting the patient three times a day, the plastic surgeon and his team were moved to say "Let us also join hands in the seva being done to this student" and waived their entire fees for the surgery.

Bhagawan and a Patient

Those were the days when Bhagawan used to accept garlands offered by devotees. Bhagawan called Sri. T.G.K. who was the district president at that time, handed over 2 garlands from the pile lying in the hall at Sundaram and directed him to deliver them at a particular address.

Bhagawan called Prof. Leelamma, the state coordinator for Balvikas, and directed her also to proceed to the same address and asked her to prepare "uppuma" - tiffin item enough for 8 or 10 people and wait there. The time given for her was hardly 1 hour.

Bhagawan reached the place at the stipulated time, entered the bungalow greeting Mrs. Hanumantha Rao "Parvathamma, ma pillanulu thesukoni ochannu. Em tiffin eppestavu?"- meaning, Parvathamma, I have brought students with me, what tiffin are you going to offer them?

Leelamma served the hot uppuma to the boys, and Swami accepted the garland that He had himself sent along with aarati just to make Mrs. Rao happy. I was a witness to this.

Where will you find a God who arranges for His garlands, tiffin, etc. just to please a devotee?

Mrs. Rao was the wife of late Sri. Hanumanth Rao, Inspector General of Prisons(IG) of the composite state of Madras. All of us have read about him in the early volumes of Sathyam Sivam Sundaram, written by Sri. Kasturi.

Mr. and Mrs. Hanumantha Rao were very staunch early devotees of Bhagawan. Swami in His teens used to visit their house very often. In fact, they had built a separate room for Bhagawan in the first floor of this bungalow. They were childless for a long time. In the late years, a boy was born to them, but he had cerebral palsy and passed away at the age of 12 years. It was Bhagawan, who filled the void for them and advised them to build a facility to treat such children. Bhagawan laid the foundation stone. The Dattattreya Orthopedic Wing of Andhra Mahila Sabha hospital in Chennai treats handicapped children, even to this day.

At the time of the current visit of Bhagawan, Mrs. Rao was ailing from hypertension and under Bhagawan's direction, I was blessed to be her attending physician and was directed to visit her daily to comfort her. I used to visit her every evening, check her BP and administer injection(B12), twice a week, and spend atleast ½ hour with Mrs. Rao. Mrs. Hanumantha Rao, who was in her 70's was living all alone in her spacious 4 bed room bungalow, had worked herself in to a depression. The doctor's daily visit was very welcome-since both were devotees and she was narrating so many stories and anecdotes of young Sathya who used to spend time with them. It was difficult to say who was treating whom? Ruminating on old happenings and memories and recounting them to a willing listener contributed to her regaining health and happiness.

For anything and everything, she wanted Bhagawan's direction. Once for her conjunctivitis, she wanted to consult Dr. Badrinath and insisted on Bhagawan's permission. There were no cell phones, those days. I had to request Sri. T.G.K. who would book a lightning trunk call to Mr. Kutumba Rao - secretary of the ashram- to convey the message to Swami. Bhagawan used to always send His blessings by the same route.

Once while she was admitted to Wellingdon Nursing Home in Chennai, Bhagawan drove down all the way from Parthi to see her and cheer her up. I was blessed to receive Bhagawan at the portico and escort Him to her room on the first floor and back.

After spending about ½ hour with the patient, the movement of the chair could be heard, I was waiting outside and opened the door for Bhagawan to step out. I could see Mrs. Rao sitting on the cot, propped up against a back rest, lamenting that she could not take padanamaskar. The compassionate Lord sat back on the chair by the cot, and raised His legs on to the cot so that she could take padanamaskar. Bhagawan was cheering her up saying "entire Madras was agog and wondering who this devotee was, because of whom, all of them were blessed to have Bhagawan's darshan". As Swami left the room, He told her, that next time He visits Madras, she has to call on Him at Sundaram, thereby assuring her recovery. As predicted, she came to Sundaram to seek blessings of Bhagawan during the following year.

A couple of years later, she had worked herself up in to a depression and was again admitted to the same hospital. A psychiatrist was called in to counsel her. After his first visit, he called me and said: "It's a simple case: she wants to meet Baba. Ask your Baba to visit her and she will be alright!!" It is easier said than done.

But Bhagawan did visit her, minutes before her passing away, a week later. Though I was not in the room, her niece who was there, reported the aroma of fragrant vibhuthi and the vertical splitting of garland placed on Bhagawan's picture opposite to the patient's bed.

Under Bhagawan's directions, she was taken to the crematorium with continuous singing by the Sundaram bhajan group.

It was a poignant moment and a learning experience to know the depth of Bhagawan's love for this devotee. I was wondering whether Swami had assured Mr. Hanumantha Rao on his anguish of leaving behind his aged wife with His well known assurance "Nenu chuskuntanu" meaning, I'll look after. Who can provide love and care like Bhagawan? We might have been fortunate witnesses to a few instances of His compassionate care… but the truth is that He cares for every being in the Universe.

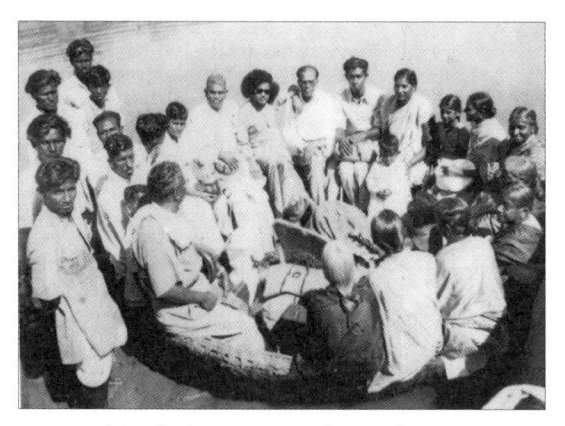

Bhagawan with His devotees on a basket boat, ready to cross river Godavari. Mrs. Hanumantha Rao, seen on far right

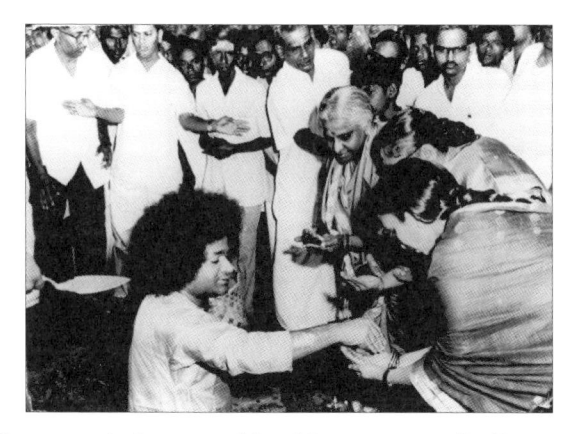

Bhagawan during ground breaking ceremony for Dattatreya Orthopedic Center of DD Hospital, Andhra Mahila Sabha, Chennai. This is an institution dedicated to serving differently abled children.

Journey via Anesthesia Practice

A six or eight year old girl, sitting in her mother's lap, was asking Bhagawan for directions one after another. Apparently Swami had presented a picture of Himself and she wanted to know whether to put it in a big frame and hang it on the wall or to put it in a small table top frame; whether it should be in her bed room, etc., etc. Bhagawan was answering all her queries patiently and in a loving tone, expressing how much He cares about her. All the time the mother was sobbing silently and not restraining her daughter. Bhagawan advised the little girl to put the picture on window sill where there is direct sun light and she can view from her study table as well as from the living room. All of us in the interview room were amazed at the loving conversation and wondered who could be this very special child!

As if to appease our curiosity, Bhagawan informed us in a soft voice that the girl's father had travelled onboard "Kanishka". Then only it dawned on us that the father of the girl had died in the tragic terror attack and the explosion that occurred onboard the Air India plane enroute to India from Canada, off the western coast of Ireland. No doubt Bhagawan was filling the void for that girl by sharing His fatherly love.

After talking to her for quite a while and giving her materialized vibhuti, Swami turned towards us and remarked "there were more than 250 passengers onboard and even if one had chanted Gayatri, the accident could have been averted." That had a profound impact on all of us.

From that time onwards, I started chanting Gayatri, whenever I travel, especially during take off and landing when most accidents happen. I gave up the habit of picking conversation with fellow passengers and instead, pray for everyone's safe journey by chanting Gayatri.

Bhagawan advises His devotees to spiritualize every activity. He has adviced housewives to cut vegetables and pray for cutting away their evil tendencies. He has said that one can roll chappathis while expanding their heart with more and more love. I was wondering what would be Swami's advise to me as an anesthesiologist.

Once it occurred to me in a flash that anesthesia is also a journey, where we take the patient by hand through stages to a mortuary like condition for surgical trespass on the body, whilst guarding from crossing safety limits. Even the slightest mishap can make the patient slip into mortuary. By definition, anesthesia is a controlled and reversible production of unconsciousness.

I always pray to Bhagawan for safety of the patient. I found that "pentothal" which we use to put the patient to sleep has to be administered as a slow intravenous injection. The time duration recommended is about 90 to 120 seconds - very long time. Just for comparison: TV channels can air 5 commercials in the same time duration.

When I timed myself, it took me roughly 30 to 40 seconds to push in 10ml of pentothal. After this particular interview, I started diluting the solution to 20ml and time the duration of injection to chanting Sai Gayatri - 3 times, very slowly. Patient's journey in anesthesia would start with this and as the Gayatri charged Pentothal permeates through blood to all cells in the body, it gives full protection and guards against any mishap.

I have had my share of challenges and complications during 32 long years of anesthesia practice. I have always felt the Divine hand protecting me and my patient as I slowly but strongly came to believe that I am not the doer but only an instrument in Divine hands. Bhagawan has put me through various experiences to confirm my belief and improve my faith in Him.

An area where the skills of an anesthesiologist are most productive and highly satisfying is the resuscitation of the new born baby. When a baby comes in to the world and is physically separated from the mother, the habitat changes dramatically from aqauatic (mother's womb) to terrestrial. Used to getting oxygen supply from the mother, the baby is suddenly denied and as it gasps and cries, the lungs open up and air enters it and the breathing process begins. The shearing stress is compared to an earthquake; however, the process happens smoothly - a tribute to God's mercy and His mysterious and beautiful creation. Very very occasionally, due to certain complications and after prolonged labour, the cry does not take place and life stands still even before it begins the earthly sojourn. At this juncture, anesthesiologist can help by inserting a tube into the baby's wind pipe and blow the lungs open - literally breathing life in to it. On several occasions, the task of accomplishing this fell on my shoulders. And each time this has been done with chanting of Sairam! Seeing a baby start its earthy sojourn with the divine name is an experience I cherish to this day.

Lessons Inside Operating Theatre

During my pre-op rounds, I saw Mrs. Mahalakshmi who was diabetic and hypertensive; and had unstable angina, 4 months before. These conditions are enough to scare any anesthesiologist.

"There is nothing to fear, is there"? She asked. It's the usual question I get asked by patients. I didn't want to scare her by explaining the risks involved in anesthesia. I told her, it is I who needs to be afraid and not her. She promptly said, Lord Venkateshwara will look after her and I should not worry about her. But she had a special request. As she was scheduled for surgery at 6:00 a.m., it coincided with her daily practice of chanting the Suprabhatham and Vishnu Sahasranamam(1008 names of Lord Vishnu). She wanted permission to bring her tape recorder and play it inside the O.R., during surgery. She was happy that her request was granted and did not have any other questions.

Promptly at 6:00 a.m., tape was turned on and auspicious chant of Suprabatham …"Kausalya Supraja…" filled the O.R. Pentathol charged with Sai Gayatri started percolating in her veins. She went under very smoothly and surgery was conducted without a hitch and all parameters monitored were within normal limits. I thanked Swami for seeing her through.

I used to say with pride that the anesthesia I administer is so perfect that my patients happily open their eyes after the last stitch is in place, awake and pain-free. But Mahalakshmi did not! She continued to sleep. Even a mild painful stimulus did not wake her up. I continued to hold the oxygen mask for her. Her breathing, pulse, B.P., were normal. Yet, she was unarousable. My pulse rate started to go up and I wondered what was wrong. My inner-voice told me to start the tape that had stopped playing during surgery. As the last line "Managalam kuru" was heard, she opened her eyes and asked me in a clear voice whether the surgery was over?

Her fixation on Suprabatham was so great that my technical skills were of no avail in waking her. The last line brought her back to consciousness. This was a great tribute to her faith in Lord Balaji and the transcendental meditation she goes into while listening and chanting the Suprabatham.

This was a great learning experience and the little ego that was left in me took a good beating!

Sujatha was a bright young girl, full of life and always cheerful. By the time she reached her 10th birthday she used to get frequent sore throat, fever, which debilitated her very much. She was found to become breathless even after walking a few yards and she complained of joint pain. Her parents had been giving her home remedies and after a few months at the suggestion of local physician, she landed in a cardiologist's office. It is here, that a diagnosis of a heart ailment was made and she was advised immediate cardiac surgery. The father who had meagre income couldn't afford the costly treatment.

She stopped attending school and her parents got her married even before her 18th birthday.

Her husband took her to a physician who also advised cardiac surgery and cautioned that she shouldn't become pregnant - delivery would be fatal for her.

Promptly she became pregnant and the mother-in-law would not permit termination of pregnancy. She wanted her grandson and not the daughter-in-law.

It was one fine morning, in the wee hours, around 2:00 a.m. I was called for an emergency C-section on Sujatha. She was already in labor for 3 hours and was in no condition to be shifted to a bigger hospital as this nursing home did not have facilities to handle cardiac emergencies.

I explained the high risk in anesthesia, given her medical history. Two lives were involved and time was running out. I gave her a sleep dose of Pentathol and 100% oxygen. As she went smoothly under, her right fist which was tightly closed relaxed completely and revealed what was in her palm: a familiar sachet of vibhuti that Bhagawan gives in the interview room. I took this as an assurance of His presence. All my tenseness vanished. It goes without saying, surgery went on smoothly and a male baby was delivered. Mother and child survived due to Bhagawan's grace.

After she recovered, I went outside to convey the good news to the anxious mother in the waiting room. She was now joined by her son-in-law. As I removed my mask to speak to them, he greeted with a Sairam! He was one of our Sevadal boys.

The mother was praying in the waiting room, I was praying inside the O.R., the patient too was praying to the same Bhagawan, without each of us knowing about it. How Bhagawan brought all of us together is a tribute to the love He has for His children and the care He bestows on them.

Whilst we remove our masks, Bhagawan seldom removes His mask He prefers to work behind the mask, unseen, unacknowledged, content in the work at hand. There couldn't be a greater lesson in humility for all of us.

Smile and be Always Reassuring

"Don't have a castor oil face and a serious look, while dealing with a patient"- is the advice I have often heard from Bhagawan. Smile and have the patience to listen to the problems, show your concern and that you care for them. Always touch a patient and talk reassuringly. Half his problems will be resolved by your empathy, never take undue risks. You should ask yourself whether you would attempt the same if he or she is your kith and kin.

"My hands are always for giving. I never ask anything from anybody. But I am asking you doctors to devote a part of your time for free seva and attend to patients who cannot afford to pay." Bhagawan said this in a discourse addressing doctors. "Kindness and compassion are tools you should use in your practice."

92 year old Meenakshi was hospitalized for a heart attack she developed while straining at stool. She was very active and otherwise very healthy. She had developed a prolapse of her uterus, obstructing urinary and alimentary passages. Her heart was perfectly normal, because of straining she developed heart attack. Now she was bed ridden. The Gynecologist was willing to do the surgery to relieve her of obstruction, but no anesthesiologist was willing to touch the patient - the risks were overwhelmingly against anesthesia.

At her prodding, her two sons who were in their 60's approached me for help. They pleaded saying they would accept the risk of loosing her on the table than to see her suffer and be bedridden.

I couldn't say no to them. She stood the surgery and anesthesia well. In half an hour, her uterus was removed and all the obstruction gone with it. A better quality of life was restored to the patient.

Saying "No" would have been the safe answer and one approved by standard practice of anesthesia; however, it wouldn't have been the compassionate answer.

This experience taught me to strive to the utmost and count on His divine mercy and grace to fulfill our compassionate efforts.

Bhagawan's Ways are Mysterious

In His master plan, He got me posted to the Cardiology dept., in mid 70's, and we were due to start the "Open Heart" unit. Until then, the only place where open heart surgeries were being done was at the Railway Hospital, Perambur, Chennai. Railway Hospital had the luxury of all the equipment and monitors; being a star dept., it attracted limitless funding from Govt. of India.

Compared to this, we at the Govt. General Hospital were least equipped. Those were early days when we had to prepare our own priming solutions. Apart from ECG monitors and defibrillators, we did not have anything - no gas analysis, and lab support was 30 minutes away in the same facility. Most of our decisions were based on our clinical acumen. With all these handicaps, cardiac surgeries had a mortality rate of 11% compared to Railway Hospital's 10%. It was early days of open heart surgery in Chennai as well as in India. Training, equipment, were a luxury due to prevailing economic conditions. Swami blessed me with an opportunity to present a paper in the Australasian congress of Anesthesiology, titled "An experience of 120 open heart surgeries without Gas Analysis".

Almost 2 decades later, Bhagawan called me and asked "Will you be able to come periodically and train our cardiac anesthesiologists in the newly built Super Specialty Hospital?" When I gratefully indicated my availability, He said: "Be ready, I will send you a telegram." I took steps to update myself and even attended open heart unit for a couple of weeks and joined in discussions and lecture classes. However, the telegram never came. I had even informed Col. Joga Rao about my readiness.

Bhagawan's ways are mysterious. He has ways of utilizing services of His devotees, not necessarily in the areas in which they have acquired skills and qualified themselves, but for the skills He wants them to acquire.

Swami sharpened my communication skills by allowing me to design and develop exhibitions on Health and Hygiene, on creating awareness on Health related topics. I had made it a point to visit various exhibits in Chennai to acquire ideas and to study display techniques, lighting, and material used for effective presentation. Later on, Bhagawan accorded me opportunity to conduct exhibition on service activities and even His life story and teachings during 2005. Bhagawan graciously visited the exhibition and took a keen interest and went through every display board in detail. During Sri Sathya Sai International Medical Conference 2005, at Prashanthi Nilayam, Swami blessed me with the chance to design the Indian section of exhibition. He also granted me the chance to be a member of the editorial team of "Sri Sathya Sai Sevadal" (quarterly magazine published from Prashanthi Nilayam) for a period of four years.

There is infinite potential inside of us. This plain truth eluded me for the longest time. Often times, we tend to pigeon hole ourselves in to our comfort zone of skills. I am grateful to Bhagawan for helping me learn that He is the doer and that with His grace, we could execute any task bestowed on us.

> "An insidious disease – unbelief – is now rampant amongst most people. It sets fire to tiny shoots of faith and reduces life to cinders and ashes. You have no criterion to judge but yet you pretend to judge. Doubt, anger, poison, and illness – all these have to be scotched before they grow. Repeat "Rama Nama"– whether you have faith or not; that will induce faith; that itself will create the evidence on which faith can be built." - Baba

Career Guidance

During 1980, by Bhagawan's blessings, I was promoted and sent to the newly built Anna Cancer Institute at Kanchipuram, Tamil Nadu. I was given the mandate to organize the Dept. of Anesthesiology, plan and equip the O.R. complex and get the surgeries started. The then Chief Minister of Tamil Nadu, was keen to inaugurate the Hospital in a couple of months and all departments were to be functional. This was a challenging task. By Bhagawan's grace I had gained similar experience in 300 bed E.S.I. Hospital in Coimbatore. I was the sole Anesthesiologist, providing services to all surgical departments for almost 1 year before a colleague joined me. The rapport that was established during this period helped me to organize the Sai Health Screening Camps in the early days.

During this period at Kanchipuram, I was commuting daily from Chennai - a one way distance of 70km, by bus. This took a heavy toll on my health, apart from the expense of spending on transport. As my children were in high school, I did not wish to relocate. Our director had promised to get me back to Chennai as the Cardiology dept. needed my services, after the new Hospital in Kanchipuram was inaugurated. As promised, He posted several candidates to replace me… however, they were influential and politically connected and none of them joined the post to relieve me. As a result, I had to drag on for 5 years.

I was at my wit's end, caught as it were, between a rock and a hard place. The daily commute, children in middle school and high school, with no alternate options materializing - this matter weighed heavily on my mind. It was during this time, Swami stepped in quietly, unasked and uninvited. He casually enquired with my son who was serving as a Sevadal in Sundaram at that time "where does your father work"? In Kanchipuram, he replied. "Oh, that is very far… 90km", Swami said. My son, in his juvenile ignorance offered, "Swami, it is 70km". "That's only in your maps" was Swami's rejoinder. The back and forth parlay did not end there… Swami expressed His concern for the long daily commute and said He was going to see what He could do. Swami approached few officials of Tamil Nadu govt. to see if I could be posted back to Chennai. That Swami would go to this extent to secure our well fare and wellbeing overwhelmed us. His motherly love and concern is to be experienced, it cannot be adequately described. However, due to circumstances beyond our control or understanding, situation remained unresolved. Perhaps, this was also part of divine drama.

The only solution I saw was to quit govt. service. This was no easy choice to make. After many sleepless nights and unable to wait any longer, I found myself waiting for darshan in Sai Ramesh shed in Whitefield. It was a Thursday and bhajans were on, non-stop. I didn't have a chance to talk to Him during morning darshan. Desperate to talk to Him, I sat the whole day in the same spot, without taking a break for coffee or lunch. Swami came for Aarti in the evening, as He was returning back to Trayee, He called me in, and I went and sat at the last row. During bhajans, Swami walked to where I was sitting and enquired as to what was troubling me. I explained what I was going through and sought His permission to quit service. He asked: "what will you do"? I replied, "Swami, with your grace, I'll take up private practice". Swami was visibly happy....He said "manchidi… chesko"(meaning: good, do it) and He lifted His robe gently for padanamaskar. The same night, I sent a letter opting for voluntary retirement and haven't looked back since.

A Course in Engineering and Management for a Doctor

It was a practice for us "Madras Trust Members" as Swami used to refer to us, to visit Parthi in the first week of December to invite Bhagawan for Sundaram anniversary(19th January). The year 2002 was no different but Bhagawan played a perfect host and spent almost two hours with us. He brought apples from inside, got them cut, and offered to all of us, followed by drinking water. He allowed spouse of trust members to join the team when one of us informed Him that ladies have also come.

When we were comfortably seated after the 'fruity' benediction, He started explaining in detail the new Japanese technology being adopted for the first time in our country for the Chennai Drinking Water Project. He explained how a thick sheet of polyethelene was being used in between concrete layers to prevent loss of water through sepage in the canal. He also explained how the automatic pavers being used for the first time in our country, would save labour, time and money with the outcomes far superior to manual paving of the canal(150km in length). Bhagawan also explained how the entire dam is being redone at Kandaleru and improving its storage capacity. He said no energy will be used in pumping water and it will be aided by gravity. He also mentioned that excess water in Krishna river that would have gone waste into Bay of Bengal can be stored and used for Chennai to solve the water problem.

When one of the trustees enquired whether this project will resolve the water problem for Chennai for the next 25, 50, 100 years...Bhagawan emphatically said: "No.... it is forever."

After narrating all the details, He explained how it was difficult for someone from Parthi to proceed to Chennai, from there to Kalahasti, and then on to project site, each time, to oversee the project. Swami then enquired very lovingly whether it would be possible for us to visit the project site from Chennai on a periodic basis(He is providing water to Chennai and is enquiring about our convenience! -that's a lesson for us in management of people and relationships). All of us said in one voice that we will accomplish the divine command. He was visibly happy. He materialized vibhuti and gave to each one of us.

Then Swami enquired if we had seen Chaitanya Jyothi. He sent for Sri. Chiranjeevi Rao. Mr. Rao who was in his late eighties arrived in no time. Bhagawan introduced him to all and requested him to telephone Sri. Bose at Chaitanya Jyothi and inform that He is sending His personal guests to be taken around. Bhagawan then enquired if our vehicles were available otherwise He would arrange a few cars to take us. We assured Bhagawan saying our cars were available and all could be accommodated.

As we took padanamaskar, He cautioned us saying "don't forget to send periodic reports to the Central Trust." No detail was missed.

He called aside Sri. G. R. Easwar(fellow trust member and long time devotee of Bhagawan) and told him not to visit the project site as it would involve a lot of walking and steep climbing. Sri. Easwar had bypass surgery a few months prior. That's His motherly love and concern.

I have visited Chaitanya Jyothi several times; in jostling crowds and as a loner. But never had experienced the joy that I did, along with colleagues and family as His chosen guests.

Chennai Water Project

Bhagawan blessed me with a chance to visit the project site 10 times in a span of 15 months. Scared of mathematics, I escaped to medicine while in school. Swami taught me what I might have missed in a engineering course, through the Water Project. It was fascinating to learn nitty gritty details and the practical working of so many aspects and the human stories behind them. After project completion, I was on a trip to project site, accompanying a Doordarshan team from Delhi. I was chosen for this mission since I could speak Telugu and be a translator for the Hindi speaking crew. We interviewed various workers. The brief for the Doordarshan team was to find out How Baba's projects are successful and completed well within a year, whereas govt. projects in five year plans always over-run on time and budget.

It was a touching experience to talk to the labour force. Most of them were from a cluster of villages in Medhak district(Andhra Pradesh) and were close relatives. They had stayed in the blistering heat(Average 50C) in the mountain region in thatched shandys, totally dependent on supplies by the L&T group(contractors) for their food and drinking water.

They had never seen Baba except in photograph. It was Bhagawan who had supplied safe flouride free drinking water to that district. Neither the British nor the Indian Govt. had solved their perineal problem of flourosis. Bhagawan had once and for all eradicated the scourge and given permanent relief. As a matter of gratitude, they toiled for Bhagawan in His efforts to provide water to Chennai. The chief engineer informed us how all of them co-operated and worked extra shifts especially when curing of the concrete had to be done continuously. He also explained: they celebrated one million man hours without any major accident or mishaps. It was his firm belief that it was Baba's grace.

Each time, we drove up to Kalahasti in the evening for a over night stay. Early morning, we used to visit the temple, do narayana seva, have breakfast, switch to company(L&T) jeeps and proceed to project site. Our main work was to record the progress by taking pictures in our cannon 35mm camera. We used to point the camera and shoot while chanting 'Sai Ram'. The following morning, film was developed in Chennai and enlarged prints were made. The results were amazing since we were not professional photographers(some of these pictures are part of Chaitanya Jyothi). The most exciting and rewarding experience would be to drive the following day to Parthi and report to Bhagawan directly, with the pictures.

This period was the most exciting and adventurous time of my life and very soul satisfying.

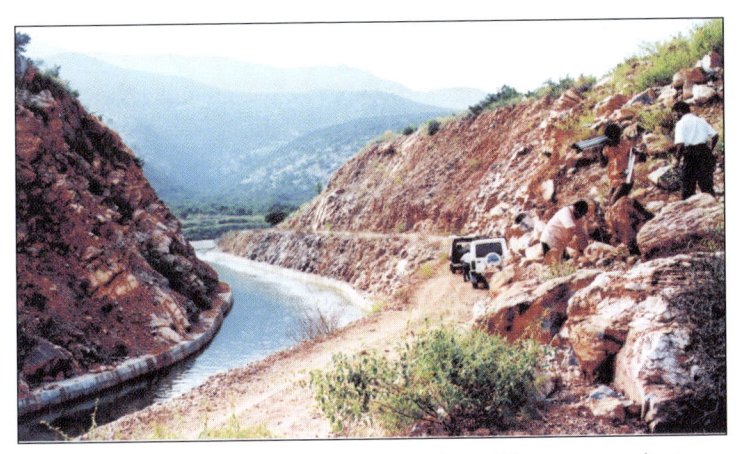

A typical scenic view of one of the sites of the water project

Red Maruti Car

My son had paid the advance for the newly announced Maruti car and we had quite forgotten about it. One fine morning we received a communication saying that we had been chosen at random to receive a car from the first batch of 300 cars made by Maruti. Being the first production batch, most of the components were imported from Japan and assembled in Gurgaon, India. In those days, one had to pay a deposit and wait for the car to be allotted.

By Swami's grace we received a red colour Maruti 800 car air lifted from Gurgaon and delivered in Chennai for Rs. 50,000, Dec. 1984. No other new car was available for this price, imported or made in India, at this time. It was a deal that was as unbelievable as it was miraculous.

It goes without saying that we first drove the car to Sundaram and placed the keys at the altar. Our first long trip was to Parthi. On our return, my son was driving. We had just crossed Ganesh gate and there was commotion along the road and people were lining up on either side. We came to know Bhagawan was expected anytime. We pulled alongside and were grateful for the bonus of extra darshan. My son had changed into a blue lungi and a coloured t-shirt. He stood away and behind the car so as to avoid being seen in that attire by Swami. Swami spotted him and pointing at his lungi had a hearty laugh. The following January when Swami visited Chennai, He mentioned to my son that Rajiv Gandhi had gifted Him with a red Maruti car. Rajiv Gandhi was then Prime Minister of India.

During this visit of Bhagawan, I had left the car at Sri. V. Srinivasan's house with a prayer that car be used for Swami or anyone of His guests. I was busy with arrangements for various programs in connection with Swami's visit. I was posted to Abbotsbury on duty one evening when Bhagawan arrived for bhajan and darshan, He spotted and told me "I thought of having a ride in your car but you are sitting here!!" I was caught on camera aghast and unable to answer Him.

Perhaps it was not right that I left the vehicle for His use without waiting and praying for it. The merciful Lord overlooked the deficiency and expressed His desire to bless my car. On the advice of my colleagues, I started waiting at Sundaram both morning and evening at the time of Bhagawan's visit to various places. Nothing happened. The last chance vanished as Bhagawan left for a short drive right after evening darshan on the day before He was scheduled to leave Chennai early in the morning… my hopes vanished in tandem as there was no other chance I could think of. I was waiting for Bhagawan's return. My car had been parked under a pandal. It had gathered a layer of dust as nobody touched it.

Bhagawan alighted from His car at the gate and walked towards the main entrance, talking and joking with devotees. Suddenly, He turned to me and said "where is your car?" I ran inside, picked up the keys and brought the vehicle to the portico. Then only, I observed the layer of dust. There was nothing I could do, Swami was waiting. As He got into the rear seat, He even remarked "Is this the way you maintain a new car" smiling all the way. He asked me to drive up to Shanti Vedika and stop. Before I realized the magnanimity of the gesture, He had alighted and was gone. I did not have the presence of mind to take padanamaskar for the boon He had granted. I was too overwhelmed for words. That is the pure love of Bhagawan and how far it stretches for the benediction of a devotee. It was like heaven with Bhagawan sitting in the rear and talking to me at the wheel. Though it hardly lasted 40 to 50 seconds, the memories of this experience is perhaps eternal… recalling this incident fills our heart with His sweet presence. His love is not bounded by time or space.

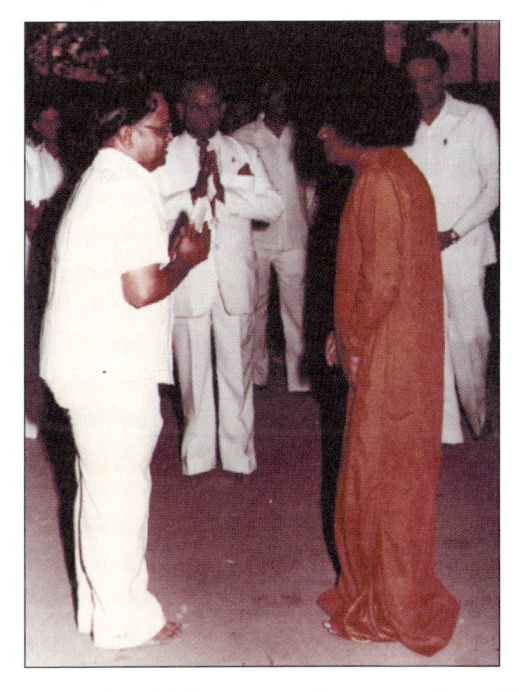

"I wanted to ride in your car, but you are here…"

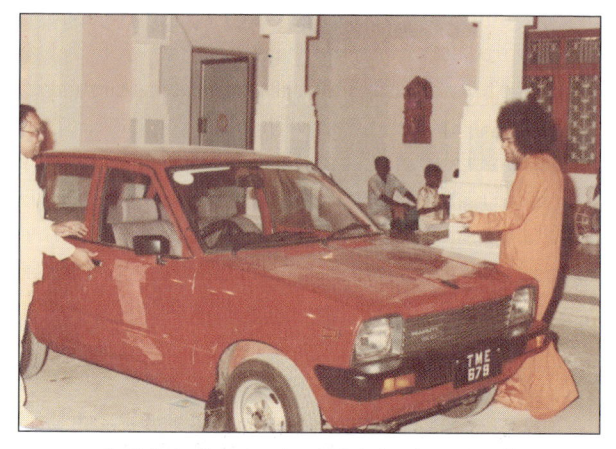

Is this is the way to maintain a new car?

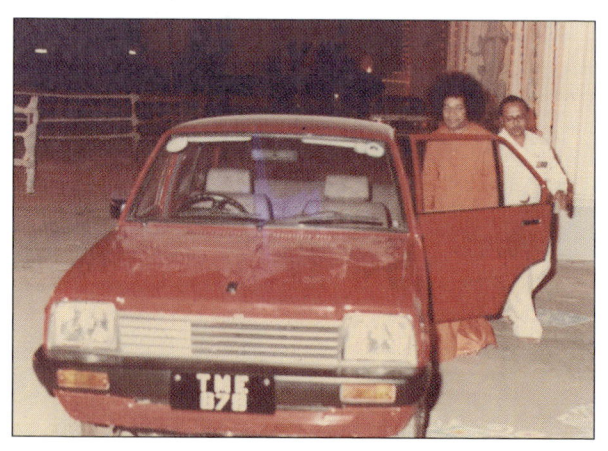

Bhagawan grants a prayer and takes a ride in the car

No Garlands for Me?

It was customary to offer garlands to Bhagawan - one on arrival, one before the discourse, and another after the discourse and before commencement of Aarati. Meticulous plans were laid out, including a roster of devotees who'd get this once-in-a-life time opportunity.

It was a lovely January evening at Abbotsbury and the atmosphere was rendered vibrant with Bhagawan's presence. A devotee had offered the customary welcome garland to Bhagawan. Bhagawan proceeded to deliver His nectarine discourse. In that discourse, Bhagawan chose to speak on garlands and flowers. He expressed His anguish that so much of money was spent on flowers for garlands and decorations. He announced that hereafter, He'd accept a single rose instead of a garland. Money should not be wasted on elaborate decorations. That was the starting point of "ceiling on desires" program introduced by Bhagawan on that day.

On that particular evening, it was my duty to offer the aarati and my colleague with the second garland was sitting to my left in the 1st row. After this announcement, his chance was lost. I proceeded straight with the aarati. As Bhagawan lighted the camphor, He made fun of me saying "You have already skipped my garland"[Photograph of this moment was captured by an alert photographer]

By this simple act, Bhagawan was modelling for us the practice of ceiling on desires. Bhagawan who is the creator of everything we use is Himself advocating for limiting the use of His seemingly limitless supply of resources. Back when Bhagawan initiated this program, conservation of natural resources had not come into vogue. Science has finally caught up with the spiritual practices encouraged by Bhagawan. Bhagawan was perhaps preparing humanity to adopt a sustainable life style in the face of rampant materialism. Climate change, waste management, which have become household words in 21st century, cannot be solved by technology alone... a spiritual life style is a necessary component of the solution. Because of Bhagawan's divine foresight and directives, Sai organization and its programs have shared this timeless message of Bhagawan on ceiling of desires with the world at large. This is our sacred task too, as those who received this Avatar's prescription have a duty to share with the wider world. In doing so, we'd be His instruments in averting a calamitous disease that humanity has invited on itself.

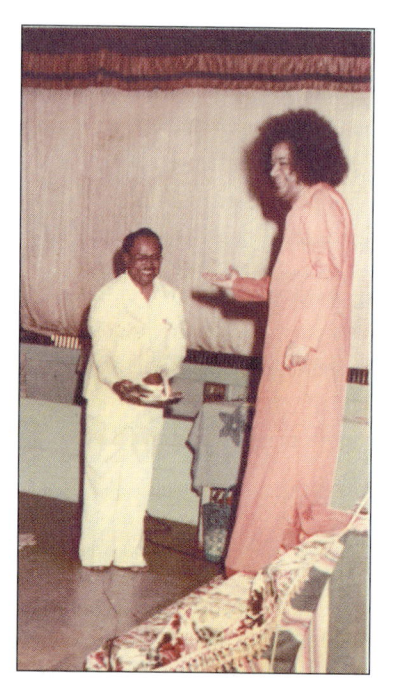

"See, no garlands for me…" Bhagawan had just finished a discourse advising devotees to curtail expenses incurred in making garlands for Swami. Swami went green long before the world woke up to sustainable practices.

Prescriptions Received During Darshan

For sometime, Bhagawan used to gather a handful of toffees from the plates brought by devotees and shower them across a large section of sitting devotees who used to gather them and partake as divine benediction - this was one more way of expressing His love from the ever giving divine hands.

At one time, myself and my colleague were seated side by side and like young children we vigourously employed our hands to catch the shower of toffees from the divine hands. In the presence of divine mother, who can help not being a child - its impossible, however old one may be. Swami smiled and told my colleague: "Neeku kadu intiki theskunu vellu"meaning: "not for you; take it home". Swami was expressing His motherly concern as my colleague was diabetic. That He remembered such a small detail about a devotee and expressed His concern instantaneously, in the midst of a large gathering, shows His immense love and care for devotees.

On another occasion I was a witness to a scene where Bhagawan had materialized vibhuthi for an old devotee and placed in his hands. The person standing behind Bhagawan offered the old man a piece of paper to safely pack the sacred vibhuthi. Swami took hold of the piece of paper smilingly, collected back the vibhuthi from the old man's palm, folded it nicely and placed it in his shirt pocket so lovingly, and touched on his head indicating His blessings. The whole act was packed with pure love and for 40 seconds, Bhagawan seemed to have nothing else to do except to concentrate on the job at hand. Perhaps, this is what Swami means by "living in the present moment" and He was expressing his love and concern for the full 40 seconds. If not for that act, neighbors sitting next to the old man would have pounced on him and plundered the benediction received by him and leaving very little or none of the vibhuthi . I have seen this happen very often. Every moment in darshan is a learning experience and His entire life has been a message for all of us.

Dorikindhi Dachuko

Seeking Bhagawan's blessings for a project, members of Sri Sathya Sai Trust(Tamil Nadu) arrived in Whitefield. We reached in the evening, just in time for bhajans and discourse. One of the students was asked to speak before Swami's discourse. What the student spoke and the way he did it, stunned everybody. He narrated an incident when during darshan, Swami asked him a straight question "what is death?"Of course the student was perplexed and dumbfounded. On His way back, Swami queried again, and after a second round, came back and gestured to him to reply. Because the student couldn't answer, Swami Himself supplied the answer stating "when I stop talking to you, it is death!" The student was no doubt awestruck. During the student's talk that evening, he tried to interpret Swami's answer and elaborate on it. He said "God is our conscience. When the inner conscience stops talking to us, it is physical death." He also explained how much Swami loves students and how well students reciprocate; and that at times, Bhagawan stops talking to them in order to correct them and the situation is worse than death and totally intolerable and makes everyone restless. The half hour talk by the student was very touching and it moved us to tears.

Next morning, after bhajans, we were called in for an interview. One of the first few questions asked by Bhagawan was "how did you like the student's talk last evening?"A proud mother showing off the achievement of the offspring. I blurted out saying "what is there Swami, they are all lucky to be trained by you." Perhaps a streak of jealously had crept into my tone. Swami retorted saying "aye..Dorikindhi daachuko". Meaning: count your blessings and be grateful. The words were sharp but delivered in such a soft and kind voice. Bhagawan did not stop with that. The mother and personification of love that He is, Swami provided me with an opportunity to serve 2 batches of MBA students whom He had brought with Him to Chennai for a visit to various industries for first hand knowledge. Some lectures were also arranged for them by the top management experts. I had the opportunity to attend classes with them as a "Sai Student." One evening, I was asked to accompany the boys to Marina beach and the famous Burma Bazzar, where you could buy imported items. After distributing pocket money to the boys, Swami called me and handed over 2 crisp hundred rupee notes and said "doctor… you also buy whatever you want." What a blessing for a pining heart which had complained to Bhagawan for having missed the chance of being a Sai student!

He also gave me an opportunity to observe at close quarters how Bhagawan organizes and manages every event so thoroughly and meticulously and in such a effortless and joyful manner - I was totally awestruck.

After the students departed in the bus, back to Whitfield, Bhagawan was to follow in a caravan of 5 cars in which He and His guests would travel. Swami gave detailed instructions as to who should travel in which car, etc., and what all things should be loaded (eatables, flask, etc.) in each of them. He wanted Mrs. Narasimhan to be seated in car #2 and Mr. Narasimhan (octogenarian editor of Sanathana Sarathi) in front seat of car #3 so that he can literally follow her. After the 5 cars were lined up, He directed our state sevadal convenor Sri. Ramani to lead the caravan in his own car, so that if there is a diversion on the way he could suggest alternate routes. Swami also directed Padmanabhan the photographer to follow Swami's car (Vehicle #5) in his own car. After Col. Joga Rao got seated in the front seat of Swami's car, Bhagawan called all the drivers one by one and gave padanamaskar and sent them to their vehicles. Just before boarding, Swami called me and said "doctor, you have not had padanamaskar and lifted His robe and gave padnamaskar" I was deeply touched by His kindness. Later on, I learnt from Sri. Ramani how he was called into Swami's bungalow after the caravan reached Brindavan, Swami supervised the lunch served to Sri. Ramani and sent him back with blessings and vibhuthi prasadam. Swami never forgets or misses anything - a great practical lesson for all of us.

This is also a form of Devotion

When the second batch of MBA students came, lodging arrangements were made at a guest house close to Sundaram so that the boys would have opportunity to be close to Bhagawan and share every meal with Him. I was put in charge of all arrangements of providing milk and fruits at night and bed coffee/tea at the guest house in the morning, stacking the fridge with ice cream and goodies for the boys to help themselves and breakfast, lunch, tea and dinner at Sundaram. No "sweet" once served was repeated another time. Prof. Anil Kumar was all praise for the feast for 1 week.

One of the boys was just recovering from jaundice and Swami used to make sure that we serve him fat free diet with plenty of fruits, etc. Bhagawan insists on all items to be served in the plate or leaf before He allows the boys to chant 'Bramharpanam'. And then, they partake the sanctified food.

One evening there was a public discourse by Bhagawan at Kamaraj auditorium(one of the biggest public halls in Chennai). I was deputed to bring the students after their industrial visit, directly to the auditorium in a special bus and accompany them back to the guest house for a wash and to Sundaram for dinner with Swami. Special seats were reserved for the students in the front 4 rows near the aisle on the right side. In the middle of Bhagawan's discourse we suddenly found, one of the students in the front row, had got up and walked to the stage and was trying to take padanamaskar. Swami had stopped his discourse, materialized vibhuthi for the student; however the student was in no mood to leave Him. Gen. Mahadevan, our state president had reached the stage from the left side before I could sprint from the right and between us we could hold the student and bring him down the stage. I quickly asked one of my colleagues to bring rest of the students to the guest house in the bus and took this boy along with me directly to the guest house. Though he was agitated, he cooperated and walked along with me to a friend's car. Bhagawan resumed His discourse. The whole incident did not take more than 90 seconds.

I brought the student with me to the guest house and because he was mentally very agitated I gave him a shot of 'compose'(tranquilizer) injection and was observing his pulse and BP closely and looking after him generally. He gradually quietened and went to sleep. It was about an hour after our arrival, Bhagawan also arrived at the guest house and came straight upstairs to see the boy. I informed Bhagawan that the student's condition was stable and he was sleeping because of the injection that was administered for calming down his agitated condition. Bhagawan smiled and informed me that "it is also a form of bhakthi" and departed long before the other students arrived. What a revelation.

At the conclusion of this trip, Bhagawan called me saying "Chalasantosham" and gave me padanamaskaram.

Seva and Service

Once Bhagawan chided me saying: "your duty does not end with handing over the pay packet at home. You run away every Sunday saying I am going for SEVA. Assisting in domestic chores and looking after children is also SEVA. In fact, it is a duty. If one does not serve at home what kind of service can one offer to society?"

Bhagawan emphasizes that when patients come in search of you to a designated place, and you offer them help it is termed as 'SERVICE'.

When you go, looking for patients who need your help and render service at their location, then it is termed as 'SEVA'.

This is the concept with which Bhagawan started the 'mobile Hospital' service in and around Puttaparthi. Villagers living in the remotest village benefit from this service.

We were able to adopt the same principle during our medical camp by doctors from all over India during Birthday festivities for a period of a week or 10 days. While our camp functions in a designated place, 24x7, we used to form a mobile team under the leadership of Dr. D. Babu and visit each shed or dormitory where devotees were lodged enquiring whether anyone needed medical help and give the medication at the site for immediate relief. Many welcomed and appreciated this service. This program was started during 75th birthday(Nov. 23, 2000) and has continued since.

Since 2015, we also have a mobile Hospital in Chennai, going around hamlets and villages with adequate facilities, offering this service over a 55km radius. Natarajan who is in his 70's from Tirupur village has this to say: "I have been suffering from tooth ache, foul smelling breath, and 3 loose teeth in my mouth for the last 1 year. My son leaves for work early morning and returns late in the night. My knee problem prevents me from going to a hospital by bus. I cannot afford to pay for the private dentist who lives nearby. Thanks to your mobile hospital: they gave me very good medicines during their first visit. This gave me very good relief from pain and foul smell disappeared. During the next visit, they pulled off all the loose teeth without any pain. Now I am able to relish food and enjoy eating. Strangely my knee pain has also disappeared."

Meenakshi, housewife from Kundrathur village is in her late 20s' and had lost first two pregnancies. Currently, during her third pregnancy, the doctor discovered that she had uncontrollable high blood pressure. He advised her frequent checkups for adjusting the dosage of medication. Because of the bed ridden mother-in-law at home, she could not visit the hospital for frequent checkup and the swelling in both her legs and breathlessness made things worse. Thanks to the mobile hospital which came very close to her house, she is able to have good treatment and her BP is under control and the swelling in the legs reduced. She is expecting her baby in a couple of weeks.

For both Natarajan and Meenakshi, the SSS Mobile Hospital has made all the difference. There are numerous such patients who feel that the mobile hospital is a great blessing from Baba. Dr. Nagaraju - director of the mobile hospital services - has been able to see perceptible change in the villages after he started teaching them about hygiene and good dietary habits.

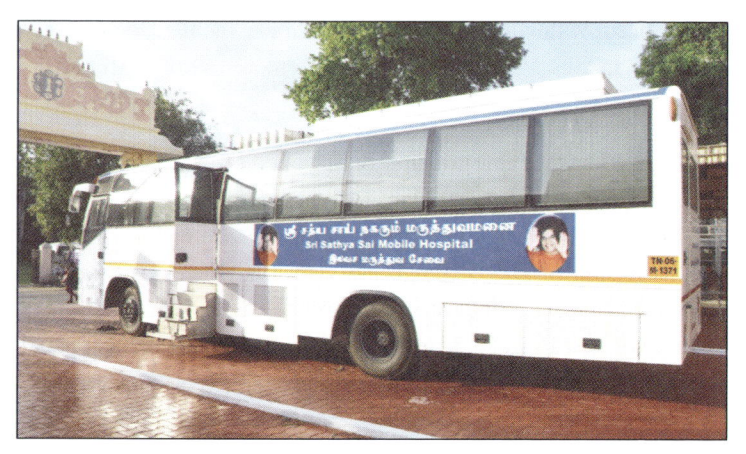

Sathya Sai Mobile Hospital, Chennai

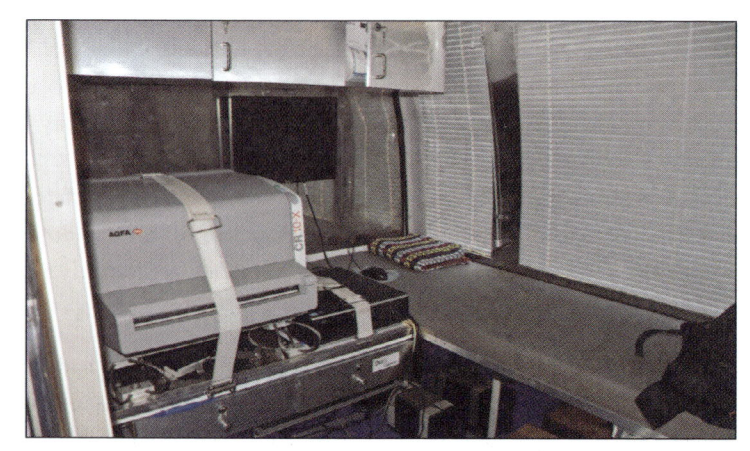

Inside view of Mobile hospital with diagnostic equipment

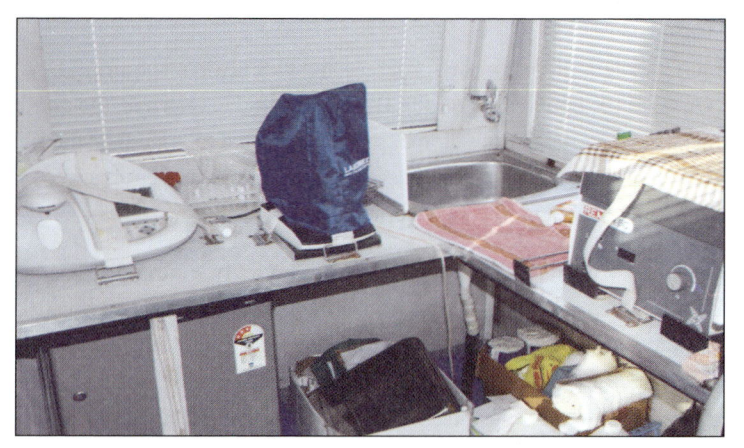

Modern clinical lab facility inside mobile hospital

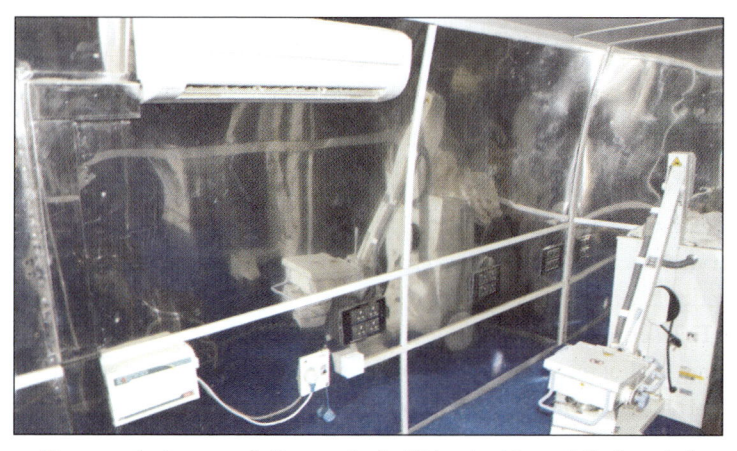

X-ray and ultrasound diagnostic facilities inside mobile hospital

You Do My Work, I'll Do Your Work

I became a free lance Anesthesiologist after taking voluntary retirement from govt. Service - I served as the Prof. and Head of Dept. of Anesthesiology at the Anna Memorial Cancer Institute in Kanchipuram, TN, India. The way this came about is a story about Bhagawan's limitless compassion that He showered on me.

Swami took a keen interest in my progress and was always enquiring how I was faring. Once, at the conclusion of our Trust meeting, He queried: "doctor, how is your practice…how much are you making"? I hesitated to announce the figure in the presence of fellow Trust members. Bhagawan smilingly remarked: "Don't worry, I will not tell the Income Tax people."

In another interview with my family, Bhagawan lovingly enquired about the rent I was paying for my apartment. When I informed him that I was paying 10,000 a month for the accommodation, He was shocked and expressed "I know, however much you make in a city, the expenses are heavy". He thought for a while and declared "Oka chinna illu vastundi" meaning: you will get a small house. A few years later, true to Bhagawan's word, we were blessed with a spacious bungalow, off Greenways Rd. in Chennai, very close to Sundaram(Bhagawan's abode and spiritual center in Chennai). In our gratitude to Bhagawan, we named the house "Sai Prema". In Bhagawan's immense compassion, He provided for my second retirement and continued spiritual sadhana.

Bhagawan has sent me to central jail, Coimbatore, several times; and Madras central prison a couple of times on His mission of Love. He has provided me endless opportunities of Seva in different locations and in different ways.

After I gave up active Anaesthesia practice due to age and health concerns, during an interview I requested Bhagawan to allot some work for me. He smiled broadly and queried back very sweetly saying: "Nenu ivalna?"meaning: should I give you work? This set a train of thoughts in my mind. Have I been egoistic in asking Bhagawan to allot me some work. How easily I had forgotten the very first lesson He taught me "look with the eyes of compassion… opportunity for seva will stare at you." It also means that any work is God's work and one has to grab every opportunity of being useful to someone or other, without waiting to be assigned some work. It also brought to mind, Bhagawan's aphorism "Duty with love is desirable; Love without duty is divine". From that moment, I have been looking for every chance of being useful and helpful. I have always given a cheering smile to every forlorn face I have encountered. The inner satisfaction derived is immeasurable.

Being involved in Sai work is a blessing that has no parallel. He has often assured us that if we do His work, He'll do our work. No earthly employer can give such a sweeping guarantee. He has taken care of my career as an anesthesiologist and has provided for me and my family in ways we couldn't fathom. He has given us the experience of the truth of His words "I'll do your work". I am forever grateful to Bhagawan for this blessing!

> "Animals did not come for the purpose of supplying food to human beings. They come to work out their own life in the world. When a human being is dead, the foxes and vultures may eat but we have not come to provide food for these that eat the human body; similarly man eats the animal, but the animal has not come to provide man with food. But we have taken to eating meat as a habit."– Baba

Divine Permission

I had the blessing of being introduced by Bhagawan on four occassions. During an interview, He had asked Dr. Bhat to join in, along with us(Trust members from Tamil Nadu, when we had gone to invite Him for Sundaram anniversary). Bhagawan introduced me to Dr. Bhat saying that I had organized many Sai eye camps at Madras and many patients had regained vision after cataract surgery. Dr. Bhat is regarded as the father of Urology in South India. He had just then joined Bhagawan's super speciality hospital at Prashanti Nilayam. Bhagawan is the embodiment of perfect leadership-it is He who inspired and provided the wherewithal for all the medical camps, nay, any and all activities; and yet, He graciously gives us the credit to motivate us to journey further towards Him.

At the completion of the interview, I was able to pick up the plastic knitted bag kept on the window sill, held it open, and followed Bhagawan as He picked up handful of vibhuthi packets and distributed to each one present in the room. After all those present had received, I held the bag in my left hand and stretched my right hand. Smiling lovingly, He picked a handful of packets and directly put them in my shirt pocket.

At that moment, I sought Bhagawan's permission to write this book on SaiKrupa experiences… He blessed me saying "Chala Santosham"(very happy). I bowed down to His lotus feet and took an extra padanamaskar.

Though I had a good collection of photographs and memories of events, I was postponing commencement of writing. When we planned SaiKrupa gratitude program as part of 90th birthday celebrations, I started to write seriously but could not complete it in time for release, on that occasion. It is divine will that the incubation period had to be prolonged-15 years had gone by after seeking divine permission.

Visiting Cards and Gifts of Love

Bhagawan accepts us for what we are and where we are, it is only we as devotees lay down conditions before we accept Him. He has to prove that He is God by fulfilling our desires-that is the main criteria. Many devotees with whom I have interacted have confessed that they started their journey in a negative way and something happened and they had a total transformation. Many male devotees have conceded that their better halves were responsible for bringing them into Sai fold. I belong to both of these categories.

I heard about Bhagawan from a classmate of mine in 1959 while at medical college. But his behaviour elicited a strong negative reaction.

During 1963, one fine Sunday, my father and a fellow judge, justice Mahajan, wanted to attend a lecture by Baba at Whites Road in Chennai in a open ground(now Sathyam Cineplex has been built at the same spot) and I was asked to drive them to the place and bring them back. I agreed on condition that I will not be asked to come inside. It so happened that for want of anything better to do, I accompanied them and sat along with them in the open ground. That day, Baba did not give a discourse, but led bhajans for a full 45 minutes. By the time the second bhajan was over, I found myself clapping and joining the chorus. It was an extremely soothing and melodious group singing led by Baba. If someone without even uttering a word could elicit pin drop silence among a 1000 people and lead them into a melodious group singing, then He must surely be worth following. The magnet started working. I was filled with inexplicable joy and happiness. In the subsequent discourses I attended, I learned for the first time that God had to be loved and not feared. That was something totally new for me.

I got married to someone who was a second generation devotee of Baba. And my wedding took place at "Sai Mandir"(Inaugurated by Bhagawan Sri Sathya Sai Baba) at Sai Baba colony, Coimbatore, India. Early morning wedding ceremony was over and preparation was on for breakfast in the temple compound. By about 8:00 a.m. a postman delivered a cover addressed to my father-in-law, having been posted from Prashanthi Nilayam the previous day.

It required courage to print "Bhagawan's picture" on the wedding invitation during those days. My father-in-law had done it and had sent the first invitation to Bhagawan. It was the practice in those days that Baba would send vibhuti prasadam as a blessing in response to the invitation.

About 4 or 5 people had taken a pinch of vibhuti before it was offered to my wife.

When she unfolded the packet, she found a enameled locket with a picture of Swami(we got it embossed in a gold frame and chain, and she wears it on special occasions). There was no way a postal cover from Prashanthi Nilayam can reach Coimbatore within a day(even today, it takes about a week). And the first delivery starts well after 10:00 a.m. on any given day. But Swami's blessings were delivered right on time and at the right place.

We had thought it was strange that bhajan was included in the program for wedding, but we were politely silent.

It was at the persistence of my father-in-law that we agreed to visit Prashanthi Nilayam as a family and seek Bhagawan's personal blessings after the marriage. More than 6 months had passed before we could accomplish the journey. The experience has been described in a separate chapter "First Encounter and Early Prescriptions."

It was during our 1985 visit when Bhagawan called us in for the first time as a family, He materialized a wrist watch for me and Himself adorned it on my left wrist. It was a square citizen watch with a gold colored strap(square dial had not yet become available in the open market). Though everybody congratulated me after the interview on being presented with a beautiful watch, it was Sri. N. Kasturi, my mentor and family friend, who cautioned me saying "watch your words, actions, thoughts, character, and heart. Doctor, Baba has given you a great responsibility and many things are expected of you - be careful." It was the most sober advice I have ever received, well before my pride and ego could raise its ugly head.

All my three children had "Aksharabhyasam" done by Bhagawan during darshan. Though they are spread all over the globe, those slates on which Swami inscribed the "Om" are taken out once a year during Saraswathi Pooja and worshipped as 'Sai Saraswathi'.

During one of the interviews immediately after our wedding anniversary, Bhagawan materialized a gold locket for my wife and pointed to her the year it was minted - 1926!

There have been many gifts of love from Bhagawan. The greatest gift is the experience of His love in our lives. My eldest son Sanjai served as Education Coordinator for the Mid Atlantic Region of USA and is actively serving, providing Sai Spiritual Education(SSE) to school age children. We live with my second son Saikiran in Chennai; he has created IT initiatives for Sai Organization of India, working with the All India President. My daughter Aparna had the good fortune to be Swami's student at Anantapur Campus. She currently serves as National youth advisor for Sathya Sai Baba organization of USA. All of us are involved in the work of Sai - this I feel is the greatest gift of love from Bhagawan, for which we are ever grateful.

He gave me an opportunity to get trained as cardiac anesthesiologist long before the super specialty hospital was thought of. He also gave me an opportunity to learn communication skills and utilize them for telling His stories and teachings. He gave me an opportunity to be associated with an engineering project.

In the early days, He blessed me with skills of event manager and which were utilized to conduct various medical camps. He also provided me with the skills and energy to conduct various seminars and conferences successfully. It is His pure love that is the pace maker for my heart which keeps beating for Him. I have had the good fortune to learn many things through many opportunities provided by Bhagawan. His love gives me confidence that He'll continue to guide to make a steady climb to His lotus feet.

When this incident happened I did not pay much attention. They had asked me whether I had visited St. Isabel Hospital the previous night to anesthetize one Mr. N. - a friend of mine. And I had denied it. 20 years later, when I read about this incidence in the book "Anyathasharanam Nasti" it struck me as a bolt from the blue. In those days, only regular panel of anesthesiologists were permitted to visit any time and administer anesthesia and new comers were not entertained at St. Isabel's Hospital. Bhagawan was obliged to adorn the garb of Dr. Vijai kumar when He rushed to the rescue of a devotee in surgical emergency. I feel quite humbled.

All of us call ourselves as tools in divine hands. Bhagawan Himself has been quoted as saying "I do not want assistants but only useful tools!" If I am asked what kind of tool you'd like to be, being from the medical field, I'll not have any hesitation in answering "surgical gloves"-which snugly fit the hands without hampering any movement and yet protecting the soft silken hands from getting soiled. Yes, then I could have the satisfaction of declaring that divine action has been accomplished through me.

Oh Lord, we should always deserve to be worthy instruments in divine hands. Jai Sairam!

Gratitude

I have no hesitation in declaring that all members of Sathya Sai Organization, including Bal-Vikas children, belonging to districts of Madras and erstwhile Chengelpet, have contributed by way of some endeavour or other in supporting the service activities at SaiKrupa in the 1980s. At that time, SaiKrupa was the main activity that involved and exposed the Sai organization to the public and media, with Abbotsbury as the epi-center. I am grateful to all of them for the guidance, encouragement, and support received by the core team.

The beauty of working in the Sai organization is the anonymity one enjoys. Many did not know my name nor did I know their names and social standing. 'Sairam' was the common greeting and the name by which we addressed each other. This helped us to focus on seva activity without any social obligations and each one gave his or her best while expressing love for Bhagawan. I am particularly grateful to Bhagawan for providing such a beautiful ambience for all of us.

Functioning of an outpatient clinic like Saikrupa, offering primary care and many specialities, and services including pharmacy and diagnostic laboratory, requires many different skills and resources. To this day, I continue to marvel at the divine providence that made this possible. Who could possibly gather all the required people under one roof in a short time? That is the power of Sai grace and blessings.

The back bone and main stay for all our programmes is the participation of enthusiastic and self effacing Sevadals and youth. They have been a great source of inspiration. Some of them have appeared in the stories and anecdotes in "Avatar's Prescription".

We were blessed to have wonderful leaders who led by their own example of dedication and devotion to Bhagawan. I am grateful for the guidance and encouragement of Sri. Damodar Rao, Sri. P.G. Achuthanandam, Major Gen. S.P. Mahadevan, Sri. V. Srinivasan, Sri. Arjuna Raja, Sri. T.G. Krishnamurthy, Sri. G.K. Raman, Sri. N. Ramani, Dr. V. Mohan, and Sri. G. Varadhan,

Bhagawan is the primal cause for this book - Avatar's Prescription. However, many of His myriad names and forms were instrumental in producing this book. I am grateful to my young engineer friend Sri. Varun Athreya of Mandaveli Samithi, Chennai. In spite of his passion for cricket and commitment to B.C.C.I., he has found the time to visit and type the original manuscript. He has shown extraordinary patience in scanning pictures for Sai archives.

Mrs. Padmini Chalikonda, an ardent devotee of Bhagawan from New Jersey, USA took on the task of drawing the sketch of Sanjeevani treatment for Lakshmana with enthusiasm and devotion. I am grateful to her for bringing to life a scene described in the holy scripture of Ramayana.

Sri. Kanakaraj - my brother from SaiKrupa most graciously took on the task of typing the original manuscript. I am grateful to him for this labour of love for Sai, and for his valuable suggestions to improve the write up.

I am thankful to Mr. Robert Mohan for promptly providing some pictures of Bhagawan from his collection.

My children have been supportive with editing tasks and numerous other small tasks that crop up every now and then in an effort such as this. I suffer from technophobia and to a large extent my children have helped me overcome this phobia to become conversant with modern tools of editing and communication. They have been honest and upfront with their constructive criticisms to help improve the book. Their mother has been a patient supporter... I am grateful for her patience as work progressed slowly but surely to what it has become today.

I am grateful to Dr. V. Mohan - my colleague and convenor of Sri Sathya Sai Trust, Tamil Nadu - for his kind and encouraging foreword for this book. In spite of his busy schedule and international commitments, he found time to review the manuscript and write a foreword.

Dr. Joe Phaneuf of USA has been very kind to go through the manuscript and offer suggestions. He also took the time to write a foreword. This speaks volumes about his deep devotion to Bhagawan and His teachings. I am deeply grateful to Dr. Joe Phaneuf.

Sri. Nimish Pandya - All India President of Sri Sathya Sai Organization - graciously agreed to write a review for the back cover, despite various demands on his time. I am grateful for his encouragement and loving support.

Like the unseen thread in the garland, Sai has been prompter, promoter, publisher, printer for "Avatar's Prescription". Like offering the water of Ganges back to the river, whilst chanting 'Gangarpanam'.... with love, reverence, and humility, I offer this book to its sacred source-our beloved Bhagawan.

Epilogue

Sri Sathya Sai Organization is perhaps the only spiritual organization where one can be a member without paying any membership fee or annual dues. It offers ample opportunity for doing seva. Even occasional visitor who wants to join in physical seva is offered an opportunity.

There are many social-welfare minded doctors and healthcare professionals who spend an enormous amount of time and effort in fund raising for their social projects. Their skills, expertise, and time is better utilized to provide much needed care. Fund raising is never a thought for the members of Sai organization due to the wonderful structure set up by Bhagawan. Necessary funds materialize on their own attracted by the pure nature of service. All of us have to be immensely grateful to Bhagawan for showing us this path. A mention must be made that while other organizations use donated funds for overhead expenses and utilize the remaining for actual service project, Sai organization is unique in applying all funds received for the service project and meeting the overhead expenses through voluntary labour of love. This is the uniqueness and sacred nature of Sai Organization.

Dear Reader, if you are a medical or healthcare professional or you just have a desire to participate in serving your community, Sai organization which dot the globe offer plentiful opportunities. No government can solve our healthcare problem. This is as much true in affluent western societies as it is in less affluent eastern societies. Its not for nothing that it was said "health is wealth". If our societies should enjoy progress and prosperity, then universal access to healthcare is a essential pre-requisite. Such universal access and availability of healthcare services can only come through service minded organizations. Sai organization under the divine leadership of Bhagawan has created a blueprint for such an organization and indeed for all of humanity. Therefore, we all have a role to play, no matter our station and profession in life.

It is much easier to write a cheque and much more difficult to give oneself to the cause of social upliftment. However, giving of oneself necessarily begets higher quality of life through self-transformation-an interesting and important byproduct of serving fellow men. This is a life that is not only aspirational but within the easy reach of one and all - thanks to the institutions and organization founded by our beloved Bhagawan. Because of this organization-Sai Organization - I had the opportunity for service for which I am ever grateful.

Dear Reader, if you are inclined or inspired to engage in service... please get involved. There is much work to be done: the cry for solace and help can be heard in every language, in every nook and corner of our planet. Bhagawan has prepared us to meet this need. Let's come together and meet this moment... and in so doing may our lives find fulfillment - that's my humble prayer!

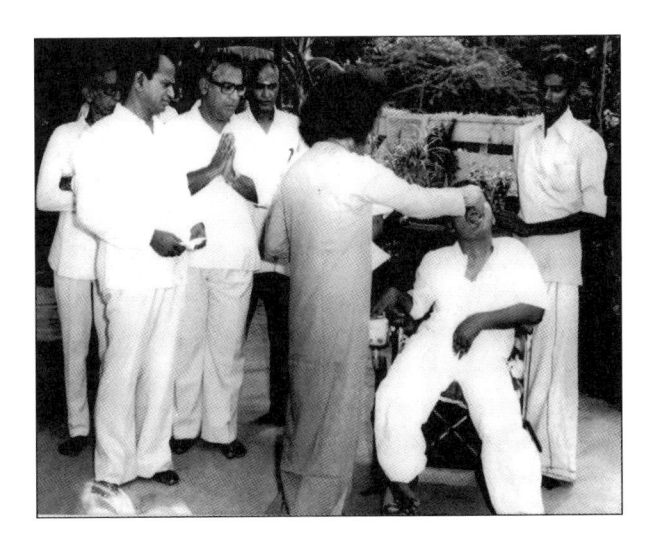